2. Oatmeal with Flaxseeds and Almonds

Ingredient:

- 1 cup rolled oats
- 1 1/2 cups unsweetened almond milk or oat milk
- 1 tbsp ground flaxseeds
- 2 tbsp sliced almonds
- 1 tsp cinnamon
- 1 tbsp maple syrup or honey (optional)
- Pinch of salt

Instructions:

1. In a medium saucepan, combine the rolled oats and almond/oat milk. Bring to a simmer over medium heat, stirring occasionally.

2. Once the oats have thickened to your desired consistency, about 5•7 minutes, remove from heat.

3. Stir in the ground flaxseeds, sliced almonds, cinnamon, and maple syrup/honey (if using). Add a pinch of salt to taste.

4. Serve the oatmeal warm, garnished with additional sliced almonds if desired.

Why this is tailored for menopause:

- Oats are a complex carbohydrate that can help stabilize blood sugar levels, which is important during menopause.

- Flaxseeds are a great source of fiber, omega•3 fatty acids, and phytoestrogens, which can help alleviate menopausal symptoms.

- Almonds are rich in healthy fats, protein, and magnesium, all of which can support women's health during menopause.

- Cinnamon has anti•inflammatory properties and may help regulate blood sugar levels.

- The sweetener is optional and kept to a minimum, as excess sugar can contribute to menopausal weight gain.

This nourishing oatmeal dish is a great way to start the day during menopause, providing sustained energy and supporting overall well•being.

3. Smoothie Bowl with Spinach and Banana

Ingredient:

- 1 cup unsweetened almond milk or oat milk
- 1 cup fresh spinach
- 1 ripe banana, frozen
- 1/2 cup frozen mixed berries (such as blueberries, raspberries, strawberries)
- 1 tbsp ground flaxseeds
- 1 tsp chia seeds
- 1 tsp honey or maple syrup (optional)
- Toppings: sliced almonds, shredded coconut, additional fresh berries

Instructions:

1. In a high•speed blender, combine the almond/oat milk, spinach, frozen banana, frozen berries, ground flaxseeds, and chia seeds. Blend until smooth and creamy.

2. If desired, add a teaspoon of honey or maple syrup to sweeten the smoothie.

3. Pour the smoothie into a bowl and top with sliced almonds, shredded coconut, and additional fresh berries.

Why this is tailored for menopause:

• Spinach is packed with vitamins, minerals, and antioxidants that can help support overall health during menopause.

• Bananas are a good source of potassium, which can help regulate blood pressure and reduce the risk of heart disease, a common concern during menopause.

• Berries are rich in phytoestrogens and antioxidants, which can help alleviate menopausal symptoms like hot flashes and mood swings.

• Flaxseeds and chia seeds provide fiber, protein, and omega•3 fatty acids, all of which can benefit women's health during menopause.

• The sweetener is optional and kept to a minimum, as excess sugar can contribute to menopausal weight gain.

This nutrient•dense smoothie bowl is a delicious and satisfying way to start the day or enjoy as a snack during menopause, providing sustained energy and supporting overall well•being.

Welcome to ***"115+ Vegan Recipes for Menopause Health and Happiness"!*** This cookbook is your comprehensive guide to navigating menopause with delicious, nutritious, and satisfying plant-based meals. Menopause is a significant life transition, often accompanied by a range of physical and emotional changes. However, with the right nutrition, you can manage these changes and maintain optimal health and well-being.

Why Vegan?

Choosing a vegan lifestyle during menopause offers numerous benefits. Plant-based diets are rich in vitamins, minerals, and antioxidants that support hormonal balance, reduce inflammation, and promote overall vitality. Additionally, a vegan diet can help manage weight, reduce the risk of chronic diseases, and improve mood and energy levels. By focusing on wholesome, plant-based foods, you can embrace this phase of life with strength and confidence.

What to Expect

This cookbook is filled with over 115 meticulously crafted recipes designed to address the unique nutritional needs of women during menopause. Each recipe is packed with ingredients that support hormone health, bone strength, and cardiovascular function. From energizing breakfasts to satisfying dinners and delightful desserts, you'll find a variety of dishes that are both nourishing and delicious.

Key Features:

- ***Nutrient-Dense Ingredients:*** Learn about the essential nutrients required during menopause and how to incorporate them into your diet.

- ***Easy and Quick Recipes***: Whether you're a seasoned cook or new to the kitchen, these recipes are straightforward and easy to follow.

- ***Diverse Flavors:*** Explore a wide range of flavors and cuisines, ensuring that every meal is exciting and enjoyable.

- ***Lifestyle Tips:*** Gain insights into managing menopause symptoms through diet, exercise, and mindfulness practices.

Empower Your Health

Menopause is not just an end; it's a new beginning. By embracing a vegan diet, you're making a powerful choice to prioritize your health and happiness. This cookbook aims to empower you with the knowledge and tools to thrive during this transformative time. Enjoy the journey of discovering vibrant, plant-based meals that will leave you feeling nourished and revitalized.

Thank you for joining us on this culinary adventure. Here's to a healthy, happy, and fulfilling menopause journey!

1. Chia Seed Pudding with Berries

Ingredient:

- 1/4 cup chia seeds
- 1 cup unsweetened almond milk or oat milk
- 1 tbsp maple syrup or honey (optional)
- 1 tsp vanilla extract
- 1/2 cup mixed berries (such as blueberries, raspberries, blackberries)

Instructions:

1. In a medium bowl, whisk together the chia seeds, almond/oat milk, maple syrup (if using), and vanilla extract until well combined.

2. Cover the bowl and refrigerate for at least 2 hours, or overnight, stirring occasionally, until the chia seeds have thickened the mixture into a pudding•like consistency.

3. When ready to serve, stir the pudding again to ensure it's evenly mixed. Top with the mixed berries.

Why this is tailored for menopause:

• Chia seeds are a great source of fiber, protein, and omega•3 fatty acids, which can help manage menopausal symptoms like hot flashes and mood swings.

• Berries are rich in antioxidants and phytoestrogens, which can help balance hormones and alleviate menopausal symptoms.

• The recipe is vegan, avoiding any dairy products that can sometimes exacerbate menopausal issues.

• The sweetener is optional and kept to a minimum, as excess sugar can contribute to menopausal weight gain.

Enjoy this nutritious and delicious chia seed pudding as a healthy breakfast or snack during menopause!

4. Avocado Toast with Hemp Seeds

Ingredient:

- 2 slices of whole•grain or sprouted bread
- 1 ripe avocado, mashed
- 2 tbsp hemp seeds
- 1 tsp lemon juice
- 1/4 tsp ground cumin
- 1/4 tsp garlic powder
- Salt and pepper to taste
- Optional toppings: sliced tomatoes, microgreens, red pepper flakes

Instructions:

1. Toast the bread slices until lightly golden.

2. In a small bowl, mash the avocado with a fork. Stir in the hemp seeds, lemon juice, cumin, and garlic powder. Season with salt and pepper to taste.

3. Spread the avocado mixture evenly over the toasted bread slices.

4. Top the avocado toast with any desired additional toppings, such as sliced tomatoes, microgreens, or a sprinkle of red pepper flakes.

Why this is tailored for menopause:

- Avocados are a great source of healthy fats, fiber, and antioxidants, which can help support cardiovascular health and reduce inflammation during menopause.

- Hemp seeds are rich in protein, fiber, and omega•3 fatty acids, all of which can benefit women's health during this transition.

- The whole•grain or sprouted bread provides complex carbohydrates, which can help stabilize blood sugar levels.

- Lemon juice and spices like cumin and garlic powder add flavor without the need for excessive salt or sugar, which can be problematic during menopause.

This simple yet nutritious avocado toast makes for a satisfying and menopause•friendly breakfast or snack, providing sustained energy and supporting overall well•being.

5. Tofu Scramble with Vegetables

Ingredient:

- 1 block (14 oz) firm or extra•firm tofu, crumbled
- 1 tbsp olive oil
- 1 cup diced bell peppers
- 1 cup sliced mushrooms
- 1 cup chopped spinach or kale
- 2 cloves garlic, minced
- 1 tsp ground turmeric
- 1 tsp ground cumin
- 1/2 tsp smoked paprika
- Salt and pepper to taste
- Optional toppings: avocado slices, diced tomatoes, chopped green onions

Instructions:

1. In a large skillet, heat the olive oil over medium heat. Add the crumbled tofu and sauté for 2•3 minutes, breaking it up with a spatula as it cooks.

2. Add the diced bell peppers, sliced mushrooms, and chopped spinach/kale to the skillet. Sauté for 5•7 minutes, until the vegetables are tender.

3. Stir in the minced garlic, turmeric, cumin, and smoked paprika. Season with salt and pepper to taste.

4. Continue cooking the tofu scramble for another 2•3 minutes, stirring occasionally, until the flavors are well combined. Serve the tofu scramble warm, topped with optional avocado slices, diced tomatoes, and chopped green onions.

Why this is tailored for menopause:

- Tofu is a great source of plant•based protein, which can help maintain muscle mass and bone health during menopause.
- Vegetables like bell peppers, mushrooms, and spinach/kale are packed with vitamins, minerals, and antioxidants that can support overall health and well•being.
- Turmeric and cumin have anti•inflammatory properties, which can help alleviate menopausal symptoms like joint pain and stiffness.
- Healthy fats from the olive oil and optional avocado can help maintain skin health and hormone balance.
- The recipe is vegan, avoiding any dairy products that can sometimes exacerbate menopausal issues.

6. Overnight Oats with Walnuts and Apples

Ingredient:

- 1 cup rolled oats
- 1 cup unsweetened almond milk or oat milk
- 1 tbsp chia seeds
- 1 tbsp ground flaxseeds
- 1 tsp ground cinnamon
- 1 medium apple, diced
- 2 tbsp chopped walnuts
- 1 tbsp maple syrup or honey (optional)

Instructions:

1. In a medium•sized bowl, combine the rolled oats, almond/oat milk, chia seeds, ground flaxseeds, and cinnamon. Stir well to mix.

2. Fold in the diced apple and chopped walnuts.

3. Cover the bowl and refrigerate overnight, or for at least 4 hours. When ready to serve, give the overnight oats a stir. If desired, drizzle with a bit of maple syrup or honey for extra sweetness.

Why this is tailored for menopause:

- Rolled oats are a complex carbohydrate that can help stabilize blood sugar levels, which is important during menopause.

- Chia seeds and flaxseeds are rich in fiber, protein, and omega•3 fatty acids, all of which can benefit women's health during this transition. Cinnamon has anti•inflammatory properties and may help regulate blood sugar levels.

- Apples are a good source of fiber, antioxidants, and phytoestrogens, which can help alleviate menopausal symptoms.

- Walnuts are a great source of healthy fats, protein, and magnesium, all of which can support overall well•being during menopause.

- The sweetener is optional and kept to a minimum, as excess sugar can contribute to menopausal weight gain.

This make•ahead breakfast is a nutritious and delicious way to start the day during menopause, providing sustained energy and supporting overall health.

7. Buckwheat Pancakes with Maple Syrup

Ingredient:

- 1 cup buckwheat flour
- 1 tsp baking powder
- 1/4 tsp baking soda
- 1/4 tsp salt
- 1 cup unsweetened almond milk or oat milk
- 1 tbsp ground flaxseeds mixed with 3 tbsp water (or 1 egg equivalent)
- 1 tbsp maple syrup, plus more for serving
- 1 tsp vanilla extract
- Coconut oil or avocado oil for cooking

Instructions:

1. In a medium bowl, whisk together the buckwheat flour, baking powder, baking soda, and salt.

2. In a separate bowl, combine the almond/oat milk, flaxseed mixture (or egg equivalent), maple syrup, and vanilla extract.

3. Pour the wet ingredients into the dry ingredients and stir just until combined (do not overmix).

4. Heat a large non•stick skillet or griddle over medium heat and lightly grease with coconut or avocado oil.

5. Scoop about 1/4 cup of the batter onto the hot surface, cooking for 2•3 minutes per side, or until golden brown. Serve the buckwheat pancakes warm, drizzled with additional maple syrup.

Why this is tailored for menopause:

- Buckwheat is a gluten•free, nutrient•dense grain that is high in fiber, protein, and magnesium, all of which can benefit women's health during menopause.
- Flaxseeds provide fiber, omega•3 fatty acids, and lignans (a type of phytoestrogen), which can help balance hormones and reduce inflammation.
- Maple syrup is a natural sweetener that is lower on the glycemic index compared to refined sugar, making it a better choice for managing blood sugar levels during menopause.
- Almond or oat milk are dairy•free alternatives that can be easier on the digestive system during this transition.

8. Green Smoothie with Kale and Pineapple

Ingredient:

- 1 cup unsweetened almond milk or oat milk
- 1 cup packed kale leaves, stems removed
- 1 cup frozen pineapple chunks
- 1 ripe banana, frozen
- 1 tbsp ground flaxseeds
- 1 tsp honey or maple syrup (optional)

Instructions:

1. In a high•speed blender, combine the almond/oat milk, kale leaves, frozen pineapple chunks, frozen banana, and ground flaxseeds.

2. Blend on high speed until the mixture is smooth and creamy, about 1•2 minutes.

3. If desired, add a teaspoon of honey or maple syrup to sweeten the smoothie.

4. Pour the green smoothie into a glass and enjoy immediately.

Why this is tailored for menopause:

- Kale is a nutrient•dense leafy green that is rich in vitamins, minerals, and antioxidants, which can help support overall health during menopause.

- Pineapple contains bromelain, an enzyme that has anti•inflammatory properties, which can help alleviate menopausal symptoms like joint pain and stiffness.

- Bananas are a good source of potassium, which can help regulate blood pressure and reduce the risk of heart disease, a common concern during menopause.

- Flaxseeds provide fiber, omega•3 fatty acids, and lignans (a type of phytoestrogen), which can help balance hormones and reduce inflammation.

- The sweetener is optional and kept to a minimum, as excess sugar can contribute to menopausal weight gain.

This nutrient•dense green smoothie is a delicious and refreshing way to start the day or enjoy as a snack during menopause, providing sustained energy and supporting overall well•being.

9. Quinoa Breakfast Bowl with Berries and Nuts

Ingredient:

- 1 cup cooked quinoa, cooled
- 1 cup unsweetened almond milk or oat milk
- 1/2 cup mixed berries (such as blueberries, raspberries, blackberries)
- 2 tbsp chopped walnuts or almonds
- 1 tbsp ground flaxseeds
- 1 tsp ground cinnamon
- 1 tsp honey or maple syrup (optional)

Instructions:

1. In a medium bowl, combine the cooked and cooled quinoa, almond/oat milk, mixed berries, chopped nuts, ground flaxseeds, and cinnamon.

2. Stir everything together until well mixed.

3. If desired, drizzle the quinoa breakfast bowl with a teaspoon of honey or maple syrup for a touch of sweetness.

Why this is tailored for menopause:

- Quinoa is a gluten•free, high•protein grain that can help maintain muscle mass and energy levels during menopause.

- Berries are rich in antioxidants, fiber, and phytoestrogens, which can help alleviate menopausal symptoms like hot flashes and mood swings.

- Nuts, such as walnuts and almonds, provide healthy fats, protein, and magnesium, all of which can support overall health during this transition.

- Flaxseeds are a great source of fiber, omega•3 fatty acids, and lignans (a type of phytoestrogen), which can help balance hormones and reduce inflammation.

- Cinnamon has anti•inflammatory properties and may help regulate blood sugar levels.

- The sweetener is optional and kept to a minimum, as excess sugar can contribute to menopausal weight gain.

This nutrient•dense quinoa breakfast bowl is a delicious and satisfying way to start the day during menopause, providing sustained energy and supporting overall well•being.

10. Vegan Yogurt Parfait with Granola

Ingredient:

- 1 cup unsweetened vegan yogurt (such as coconut, almond, or soy•based)
- 1/2 cup fresh or frozen berries (such as blueberries, raspberries, or strawberries)
- 1/4 cup homemade or store•bought granola (without added sugars)
- 1 tbsp chia seeds or ground flaxseeds
- 1 tsp honey or maple syrup (optional)

Instructions:

1. In a parfait glass or bowl, layer the vegan yogurt, fresh or frozen berries, and granola.

2. Sprinkle the chia seeds or ground flaxseeds over the top.

3. If desired, drizzle a teaspoon of honey or maple syrup over the parfait.

4. Serve chilled and enjoy!

Why this is tailored for menopause:

- Vegan yogurt is a dairy•free, probiotic•rich option that can be easier on the digestive system during menopause.

- Berries are packed with antioxidants, fiber, and phytoestrogens, which can help alleviate menopausal symptoms like hot flashes and mood swings.

- Granola provides complex carbohydrates and fiber to help maintain steady energy levels, without the added sugars that can be problematic during menopause.

- Chia seeds and flaxseeds are excellent sources of fiber, protein, and omega•3 fatty acids, all of which can benefit women's health during this transition.

- The sweetener is optional and kept to a minimum, as excess sugar can contribute to menopausal weight gain.

This layered vegan yogurt parfait is a delicious and nutritious breakfast or snack that can help support overall well•being during menopause. The combination of probiotics, antioxidants, and fiber•rich ingredients makes it a great choice for this stage of life.

11. Roasted Chickpeas

Ingredient:

- 1 (15 oz) can of chickpeas, drained and rinsed
- 1 tbsp olive oil
- 1 tsp ground cumin
- 1 tsp paprika
- 1/2 tsp garlic powder
- 1/4 tsp cayenne pepper (optional)
- 1/2 tsp sea salt

Instructions:

1. Preheat your oven to 400°F (200°C).

2. Pat the drained and rinsed chickpeas dry with a paper towel or clean kitchen towel.

3. In a medium bowl, toss the chickpeas with the olive oil, cumin, paprika, garlic powder, and cayenne pepper (if using). Sprinkle with sea salt and mix well to coat the chickpeas evenly.

4. Spread the seasoned chickpeas in a single layer on a baking sheet lined with parchment paper.

5. Roast the chickpeas in the preheated oven for 20•25 minutes, stirring halfway, until they are crispy and golden brown.

6. Remove the roasted chickpeas from the oven and let them cool for a few minutes before serving.

Why this is tailored for menopause:

- Chickpeas are a great source of plant•based protein, fiber, and complex carbohydrates, which can help maintain energy levels and blood sugar balance during menopause.

- The spices used, such as cumin, paprika, and garlic powder, have anti•inflammatory properties that can help alleviate menopausal symptoms like joint pain and stiffness.

Roasted chickpeas are a versatile, nutrient•dense snack that can be enjoyed on their own or as a topping for salads, soups, or other dishes during menopause. They provide a satisfying crunch and a boost of plant•based protein and fiber.

12. Edamame with Sea Salt

Ingredient:

- 1 lb frozen edamame in the pod
- 1 tsp sea salt

Instructions:

1. Bring a large pot of water to a boil.

2. Add the frozen edamame pods to the boiling water and cook for 5•7 minutes, until the pods are bright green and tender.

3. Drain the edamame and transfer to a serving bowl.

4. Sprinkle the sea salt over the hot edamame and toss to coat evenly.

5. Serve the edamame warm, with the pods intact. Encourage guests to pop the edamame beans out of the pods with their teeth.

Why this is tailored for menopause:

- Edamame is a great source of plant•based protein, fiber, and isoflavones (a type of phytoestrogen), all of which can benefit women's health during menopause.

- The isoflavones in edamame may help alleviate menopausal symptoms like hot flashes and mood swings.

- Sea salt provides a simple, flavorful seasoning without the need for added sugars or unhealthy fats.

- This snack is vegan, making it suitable for those who may be avoiding animal products during menopause.

- Edamame is a low•calorie, nutrient•dense option that can help with weight management, a common concern during the menopausal transition.

Edamame with sea salt is a quick, easy, and menopause•friendly snack that can be enjoyed as a healthy appetizer or side dish. The combination of protein, fiber, and phytoestrogens makes it a great choice for supporting overall well•being during menopause.

13. Hummus with Veggie Sticks

Ingredient:

- 1 (15 oz) can of chickpeas, drained and rinsed
- 2 tbsp tahini
- 2 tbsp fresh lemon juice
- 1 clove garlic, minced
- 2 tbsp olive oil
- 1/4 tsp ground cumin
- 1/4 tsp paprika
- Salt and pepper to taste
- Assorted veggie sticks (such as carrots, celery, cucumber, bell peppers)

Instructions:

1. In a food processor or high•speed blender, combine the drained and rinsed chickpeas, tahini, lemon juice, minced garlic, olive oil, cumin, and paprika. Blend until smooth and creamy.

2. Season the hummus with salt and pepper to taste. Transfer the hummus to a serving bowl and serve with an assortment of fresh veggie sticks, such as carrot, celery, cucumber, and bell pepper slices.

Why this is tailored for menopause:

- Chickpeas are a great source of plant•based protein, fiber, and complex carbohydrates, which can help maintain energy levels and blood sugar balance during menopause.
- Tahini is rich in calcium, which is important for bone health during this transition.

- Lemon juice and spices like cumin and paprika have anti•inflammatory properties that can help alleviate menopausal symptoms like joint pain and stiffness.

- The vegetables provide a variety of vitamins, minerals, and antioxidants that can support overall health and well•being during menopause.

- This recipe is vegan, making it suitable for those who may be avoiding animal products during this stage of life.

Hummus with fresh veggie sticks is a nutritious and satisfying snack that can help support overall health and well•being during menopause. The combination of plant•based protein, fiber, and anti•inflammatory ingredients makes it a great choice for this transition.

14. Almond Butter on Rice Cakes

Ingredient:

- 2 whole grain or brown rice cakes
- 2 tbsp natural almond butter
- 1 tsp chia seeds (optional)
- 1/4 tsp ground cinnamon (optional)

Instructions:

1. Spread the almond butter evenly over the rice cakes.

2. If desired, sprinkle the chia seeds and ground cinnamon over the almond butter.

That's it! This simple snack is ready to enjoy.

Why this is tailored for menopause:

• Rice cakes provide a gluten•free, complex carbohydrate base that can help maintain steady energy levels during menopause.

• Almond butter is a great source of healthy fats, protein, and magnesium, all of which can support overall health and well•being during this transition.

• Chia seeds are rich in fiber, protein, and omega•3 fatty acids, which can help manage menopausal symptoms like hot flashes and mood swings.

• Cinnamon has anti•inflammatory properties and may help regulate blood sugar levels, which can be beneficial during menopause.

• This snack is vegan, making it suitable for those who may be avoiding animal products during this stage of life.

• The simplicity of the recipe allows the natural flavors of the almond butter and rice cakes to shine, without the need for added sugars or unhealthy fats.

Almond butter on rice cakes is a quick, easy, and nutritious snack that can help satisfy hunger and provide sustained energy during menopause. The combination of healthy fats, complex carbohydrates, and optional superfoods makes it a great choice for supporting overall well•being.

15. Fruit Salad with Mint

Ingredient:

- 1 cup diced watermelon
- 1 cup diced pineapple
- 1 cup diced strawberries
- 1 cup blueberries
- 2 tbsp freshly chopped mint leaves
- 1 tbsp lime juice
- 1 tsp honey or maple syrup (optional)

Instructions:

1. In a large bowl, combine the diced watermelon, pineapple, strawberries, and blueberries.

2. Add the freshly chopped mint leaves and drizzle the lime juice over the fruit.

3. If desired, drizzle a teaspoon of honey or maple syrup over the fruit salad for a touch of sweetness.

4. Gently toss the fruit salad to combine all the ingredients. Serve the fruit salad chilled or at room temperature.

Why this is tailored for menopause:

- Watermelon is a hydrating fruit that is rich in vitamins, minerals, and antioxidants, which can help support overall health during menopause.

- Pineapple contains bromelain, an enzyme with anti•inflammatory properties, which can help alleviate menopausal symptoms like joint pain and stiffness.

- Strawberries and blueberries are packed with antioxidants, fiber, and phytoestrogens, which can help balance hormones and reduce the frequency and intensity of hot flashes.

- Mint leaves have a refreshing flavor and can help soothe digestive issues, which can sometimes be a concern during menopause.

This vibrant and refreshing fruit salad is a great way to incorporate a variety of nutrient•dense fruits into your diet during menopause, providing hydration, antioxidants, and anti•inflammatory benefits.

16. Kale Chips

Ingredient:

- 1 bunch of kale, stems removed and leaves torn into bite•sized pieces
- 1 tbsp olive oil
- 1 tsp sea salt
- 1/2 tsp garlic powder (optional)
- 1/4 tsp cayenne pepper (optional)

Instructions:

1. Preheat your oven to 325°F (165°C).

2. Wash and thoroughly dry the kale leaves. Tear or cut the leaves into bite•sized pieces, discarding the tough stems.

3. In a large bowl, toss the kale leaves with the olive oil, sea salt, and any optional seasonings (garlic powder, cayenne pepper).

4. Spread the kale leaves in a single layer on one or more baking sheets, making sure they are not overlapping.

5. Bake the kale chips in the preheated oven for 12•15 minutes, flipping them halfway, until they are crispy and lightly browned. Remove the kale chips from the oven and let them cool for a few minutes before serving.

Why this is tailored for menopause:

- Kale is a nutrient•dense leafy green that is rich in vitamins, minerals, and antioxidants, which can help support overall health during menopause.

- The optional seasonings, such as garlic powder and cayenne pepper, have anti•inflammatory properties that can help alleviate menopausal symptoms like joint pain and stiffness.

- Cayenne pepper contains capsaicin, which may help reduce the frequency and intensity of hot flashes.

Kale chips are a versatile, nutrient•dense snack that can be enjoyed during menopause. The combination of vitamins, minerals, and anti•inflammatory properties makes them a great choice for supporting overall well•being during this transition.

17. Energy Balls with Dates and Nuts

Ingredient:

- 1 cup pitted Medjool dates
- 1/2 cup raw almonds or walnuts
- 2 tbsp ground flaxseeds
- 1 tbsp unsweetened shredded coconut
- 1 tsp ground cinnamon
- 1/4 tsp sea salt

Instructions:

1. In a food processor, blend the pitted Medjool dates until they form a sticky, paste•like consistency.

2. Add the raw almonds or walnuts, ground flaxseeds, shredded coconut, cinnamon, and sea salt to the food processor. Pulse until the mixture is well combined and starts to form a dough•like consistency.

3. Scoop out tablespoon•sized portions of the mixture and roll them into bite•sized balls with your hands.

4. Place the energy balls on a parchment•lined baking sheet and refrigerate for at least 30 minutes to allow them to firm up.

5. Serve the energy balls chilled or at room temperature. Store any leftovers in an airtight container in the refrigerator for up to 1 week.

Why this is tailored for menopause:

- Dates are a natural source of fiber, vitamins, and minerals, which can help maintain energy levels and digestive health during menopause.

- Nuts, such as almonds and walnuts, provide healthy fats, protein, and magnesium, all of which can support overall well•being during this transition.

- Flaxseeds are a great source of fiber, omega•3 fatty acids, and lignans (a type of phytoestrogen), which can help balance hormones and reduce inflammation.

These delicious and wholesome energy balls are a great way to fuel your body during menopause, supporting overall health and well•being.

18. Trail Mix with Seeds and Dried Fruits

Ingredient:

- 1/2 cup raw unsalted pumpkin seeds
- 1/2 cup raw unsalted sunflower seeds
- 1/2 cup raw unsalted almonds
- 1/2 cup unsweetened dried cranberries
- 1/2 cup unsweetened dried apricots, chopped
- 2 tbsp chia seeds
- 1 tsp ground cinnamon (optional)

Instructions:

1. In a large bowl, combine the pumpkin seeds, sunflower seeds, almonds, dried cranberries, dried apricots, and chia seeds.

2. If desired, sprinkle the ground cinnamon over the trail mix and stir to distribute evenly.

3. Transfer the trail mix to an airtight container or resealable bag. Store at room temperature for up to 2 weeks.

Why this is tailored for menopause:

- Pumpkin seeds and sunflower seeds are rich in zinc, magnesium, and antioxidants, which can help support immune function and bone health during menopause.

- Almonds provide healthy fats, protein, and magnesium, all of which can benefit women's health during this transition.

- Dried cranberries and apricots are good sources of fiber, vitamins, and phytoestrogens, which can help alleviate menopausal symptoms like hot flashes and mood swings.

- Chia seeds are a great source of fiber, protein, and omega•3 fatty acids, which can help manage menopausal symptoms and support overall well•being.

- Cinnamon has anti•inflammatory properties and may help regulate blood sugar levels, which can be beneficial during menopause.

This nutrient•dense trail mix is a convenient and portable snack that can help provide sustained energy, support bone health, and alleviate menopausal symptoms. Enjoy it as a midday pick•me•up or as a healthy addition to your daily routine during menopause.

19. Apple Slices with Peanut Butter

Ingredient:

- 1 medium apple, cored and sliced
- 2 tbsp natural peanut butter (or almond butter)
- 1 tsp ground cinnamon (optional)

Instructions:

1. Wash and slice the apple into thin wedges or slices.

2. Spread a small amount of peanut butter (or almond butter) onto each apple slice.

3. If desired, sprinkle a light dusting of ground cinnamon over the peanut butter•topped apple slices.

Why this is tailored for menopause:

- Apples are a good source of fiber, antioxidants, and phytoestrogens, which can help alleviate menopausal symptoms like hot flashes and mood swings.

- Peanut butter (or almond butter) provides healthy fats, protein, and magnesium, all of which can support overall health during menopause.

- Cinnamon has anti•inflammatory properties and may help regulate blood sugar levels, which can be beneficial during this transition.

- This snack is vegan, making it suitable for those who may be avoiding animal products during menopause.

- The simplicity of the recipe allows the natural flavors of the apple and nut butter to shine, without the need for added sugars or unhealthy fats.

Apple slices with peanut butter (or almond butter) make for a quick, easy, and nutritious snack that can help satisfy hunger and provide sustained energy during menopause. The combination of fiber, healthy fats, and antioxidants makes it a great choice for supporting overall well•being.

20. Dark Chocolate and Almonds

Ingredient:

- 1 oz dark chocolate (70% cacao or higher), chopped
- 1/4 cup raw unsalted almonds

Instructions:

1. In a small bowl, combine the chopped dark chocolate and raw almonds.

That's it! This simple snack is ready to enjoy.

Why this is tailored for menopause:

- Dark chocolate (70% cacao or higher) is rich in antioxidants and may help improve mood and cognitive function, which can be beneficial during menopause.

- Almonds are a great source of healthy fats, protein, and magnesium, all of which can support overall health and well•being during this transition.

- This snack is vegan, making it suitable for those who may be avoiding animal products during menopause.

- The simplicity of the recipe allows the natural flavors of the dark chocolate and almonds to shine, without the need for added sugars or unhealthy fats.

Dark chocolate and almonds make for a satisfying and nutrient•dense snack that can help satisfy cravings and provide a boost of energy during menopause. The combination of antioxidants, healthy fats, and minerals makes it a great choice for supporting overall well•being during this stage of life.

Remember to enjoy this snack in moderation, as dark chocolate and nuts can be high in calories. Portion control is key for maintaining a healthy weight during menopause.

21. Lentil Soup with Spinach

Ingredient:

- 1 cup dry brown or green lentils, rinsed
- 4 cups low•sodium vegetable broth
- 1 tbsp olive oil
- 1 onion, diced
- 2 carrots, peeled and diced
- 2 celery stalks, diced
- 3 garlic cloves, minced
- 1 tsp ground cumin
- 1 tsp dried thyme
- 1/4 tsp cayenne pepper (optional)
- Salt and pepper to taste
- 2 cups fresh spinach, chopped

Instructions:

1. In a large pot, combine the rinsed lentils and vegetable broth. Bring to a boil over high heat, then reduce heat and simmer for 15•20 minutes, until the lentils are tender.

2. In a separate skillet, heat the olive oil over medium heat. Add the diced onion, carrots, and celery. Sauté for 5•7 minutes, until the vegetables are softened.

3. Add the minced garlic, cumin, thyme, and cayenne pepper (if using) to the sautéed vegetables. Cook for 1•2 minutes, until fragrant.

4. Transfer the sautéed vegetable mixture to the pot with the cooked lentils. Stir to combine. Season the lentil soup with salt and pepper to taste. Just before serving, stir in the chopped fresh spinach and allow it to wilt in the hot soup. Serve the lentil soup warm.

Why this is tailored for menopause:

• Lentils are a great source of plant•based protein, fiber, and complex carbohydrates, which can help maintain energy levels and blood sugar balance during menopause.

• Spinach is a nutrient•dense leafy green that provides vitamins, minerals, and antioxidants to support overall health.

This hearty and nourishing lentil soup with spinach is a delicious and menopause•friendly meal that provides a balance of plant•based protein, fiber, and anti•inflammatory ingredients to support overall well•being.

22. Quinoa Salad with Chickpeas and Avocado

Ingredient:

- 1 cup cooked quinoa, cooled
- 1 (15 oz) can chickpeas, drained and rinsed
- 1 avocado, diced
- 1 cup cherry tomatoes, halved
- 1/2 cup diced cucumber
- 1/4 cup chopped red onion
- 2 tbsp chopped fresh parsley
- 2 tbsp olive oil
- 2 tbsp lemon juice
- 1 tsp Dijon mustard
- 1/2 tsp ground cumin
- Salt and pepper to taste

Instructions:

1. In a large bowl, combine the cooked and cooled quinoa, drained and rinsed chickpeas, diced avocado, cherry tomatoes, diced cucumber, chopped red onion, and chopped parsley.

2. In a small bowl, whisk together the olive oil, lemon juice, Dijon mustard, and ground cumin. Season the dressing with salt and pepper to taste.

3. Pour the dressing over the quinoa salad and gently toss to coat all the ingredients. Serve the Quinoa Salad with Chickpeas and Avocado chilled or at room temperature.

Why this is tailored for menopause:

- Quinoa is a gluten•free, high•protein grain that can help maintain energy levels and muscle mass during menopause.

- Chickpeas are a great source of plant•based protein, fiber, and complex carbohydrates, which can help stabilize blood sugar levels.

- Avocado provides healthy fats, fiber, and antioxidants that can support cardiovascular health and reduce inflammation during this transition.

This colorful and nutrient•dense quinoa salad is a delicious and satisfying meal or side dish that can support overall well•being during menopause, providing a balance of complex carbohydrates, protein, healthy fats, and anti•inflammatory ingredients.

23. Buddha Bowl with Sweet Potato and Tahini

Ingredient:

- 1 medium sweet potato, peeled and cubed
- 1 cup cooked quinoa
- 1 cup shredded kale or spinach
- 1/2 cup cooked chickpeas
- 2 tbsp tahini
- 1 tbsp lemon juice
- 1 tbsp water
- Salt and pepper to taste
- Optional toppings: avocado, roasted vegetables, toasted nuts/seeds

Instructions:

1. Preheat oven to 400°F. Toss the cubed sweet potato with a drizzle of olive oil and season with salt and pepper. Roast for 20•25 minutes, until tender.

2. In a small bowl, whisk together the tahini, lemon juice, and water to make a tahini dressing. Season with salt and pepper.

3. In a large bowl, combine the roasted sweet potato, quinoa, kale/spinach, and chickpeas.

4. Drizzle the tahini dressing over the bowl and toss gently to coat.

5. Top with any additional desired toppings like avocado, roasted veggies, toasted nuts or seeds.

6. Serve immediately and enjoy your nourishing Buddha bowl!

24. Vegan Caesar Salad with Tofu

Ingredient:

Salad:
- 5 cups chopped romaine lettuce
- 1 cup cubed extra•firm tofu
- 1/2 cup croutons (optional)

Dressing:
- 1/2 cup raw cashews, soaked in water for at least 4 hours or overnight
- 1/4 cup unsweetened almond milk
- 2 tbsp fresh lemon juice
- 1 tbsp Dijon mustard
- 1 garlic clove, minced
- 1 tsp capers (optional)
- 1/4 tsp sea salt
- 1/4 tsp black pepper

Instructions:

1. Drain and rinse the soaked cashews. In a high•speed blender, combine the cashews, almond milk, lemon juice, Dijon mustard, garlic, capers (if using), salt, and pepper. Blend until smooth and creamy. Set the dressing aside.

2. In a large salad bowl, combine the chopped romaine lettuce and cubed tofu. Drizzle the vegan Caesar dressing over the salad and toss gently to coat.

3. Top the salad with croutons, if desired. Serve the Vegan Caesar Salad with Tofu immediately.

Why this is tailored for menopause:

- Romaine lettuce is a nutrient•dense leafy green that provides vitamins, minerals, and antioxidants to support overall health during menopause.

- Tofu is a great source of plant•based protein, which can help maintain muscle mass and energy levels during this transition.

- Cashews in the dressing provide healthy fats and minerals like magnesium, which can benefit women's health during menopause.

This Vegan Caesar Salad with Tofu is a nutritious and satisfying meal that can help support overall well•being during menopause, providing a balance of protein, fiber, and anti•inflammatory ingredients.

25. Black Bean and Corn Salad

Ingredient:

- 1 (15 oz) can black beans, drained and rinsed
- 1 (15 oz) can corn, drained
- 1 cup cherry tomatoes, halved
- 1/2 red onion, diced
- 1 avocado, diced
- 1/4 cup chopped cilantro
- 2 tbsp lime juice
- 1 tbsp olive oil
- 1 tsp cumin
- 1/2 tsp chili powder
- Salt and pepper to taste

Instructions:

1. In a large bowl, combine the drained and rinsed black beans, drained corn, halved cherry tomatoes, diced red onion, and diced avocado.

2. Add the chopped cilantro, lime juice, olive oil, cumin, and chili powder. Toss everything together until well combined.

3. Season with salt and pepper to taste.

4. Refrigerate the salad for at least 30 minutes to allow the flavors to meld together.

5. Serve chilled or at room temperature. This salad makes a great side dish or can be enjoyed on its own as a light main course.

Enjoy your fresh and flavorful Black Bean and Corn Salad!

26. Stuffed Bell Peppers with Brown Rice

Ingredient:

- 4 medium bell peppers, halved and seeded
- 1 cup cooked brown rice
- 1 (15 oz) can black beans, drained and rinsed
- 1 cup diced tomatoes
- 1/2 cup diced onion
- 2 cloves garlic, minced
- 1 tsp ground cumin
- 1 tsp dried oregano
- 1/4 tsp cayenne pepper (optional)
- Salt and pepper to taste
- 1/4 cup shredded vegan cheese (optional)

Instructions:

1. Preheat your oven to 375°F (190°C).

2. Arrange the bell pepper halves in a baking dish or on a rimmed baking sheet.

3. In a medium bowl, combine the cooked brown rice, black beans, diced tomatoes, onion, garlic, cumin, oregano, and cayenne pepper (if using). Season with salt and pepper to taste.

4. Spoon the rice and bean mixture evenly into the bell pepper halves.

5. If using, sprinkle the shredded vegan cheese over the top of the stuffed peppers.

6. Bake the stuffed peppers in the preheated oven for 25•30 minutes, or until the peppers are tender and the filling is heated through. Serve the stuffed bell peppers warm.

Why this is tailored for menopause:

- Bell peppers are a good source of vitamins, minerals, and antioxidants, which can support overall health during menopause.

- Brown rice provides complex carbohydrates, fiber, and B vitamins, which can help maintain energy levels and blood sugar balance.

These colorful and nutrient•dense stuffed bell peppers make for a satisfying and menopause•friendly main dish or side, providing a balance of complex carbohydrates, protein, and anti•inflammatory ingredients.

27. Falafel Wrap with Hummus

Ingredient:

- 1 (15 oz) can chickpeas, drained and rinsed
- 1/2 cup fresh parsley, chopped
- 1/4 cup fresh cilantro, chopped
- 2 cloves garlic, minced
- 1 tsp ground cumin
- 1/2 tsp ground coriander
- 1/4 tsp cayenne pepper
- 2 tbsp whole wheat flour
- Salt and pepper to taste
- 2 tbsp olive oil
- 4 whole wheat tortillas or pita breads
- 1 cup hummus
- 1 cup mixed greens
- 1/2 cup diced cucumber
- 1/4 cup diced red onion

Instructions:

1. In a food processor, combine the drained chickpeas, parsley, cilantro, garlic, cumin, coriander, and cayenne. Pulse until a coarse paste forms.

2. Transfer the chickpea mixture to a bowl and stir in the whole wheat flour. Season with salt and pepper.

3. Form the mixture into small falafel balls, about 1•2 tablespoons each.

4. In a skillet, heat the olive oil over medium heat. Fry the falafel balls for 2•3 minutes per side until golden brown.

5. Spread a layer of hummus onto each tortilla or pita. Top with the fried falafel, mixed greens, diced cucumber, and red onion.

6. Wrap or fold the tortilla/pita around the fillings and enjoy!

This falafel wrap is packed with plant•based protein, fiber, and nutrients that can help support women during menopause. The chickpeas, hummus, and vegetables provide a balanced, nourishing meal.

28. Vegan Sushi Rolls with Avocado

Ingredient:

- 1 cup short•grain brown rice, cooked according to package instructions
- 2 tbsp rice vinegar
- 1 tsp maple syrup or honey
- 1/4 tsp sea salt
- 1 avocado, sliced
- 1 cucumber, peeled and cut into thin strips
- 1 carrot, peeled and cut into thin strips
- Nori sheets
- Sesame seeds (optional)

Instructions:

1. In a medium bowl, combine the cooked brown rice, rice vinegar, maple syrup or honey, and sea salt. Stir until well mixed.

2. Lay a nori sheet shiny•side down on a sushi mat or clean surface. Spread about 1/2 cup of the seasoned rice evenly over the nori, leaving a 1•inch border at the top.

3. Arrange the avocado, cucumber, and carrot strips in a line across the center of the rice.

4. Carefully roll the nori sheet tightly around the fillings, using the sushi mat to help you. Moisten the top edge of the nori with a bit of water to seal the roll.

5. Slice the sushi roll into 6•8 pieces using a sharp, wet knife. Repeat the process with the remaining nori sheets and fillings. Serve the vegan sushi rolls garnished with sesame seeds, if desired.

Why this is tailored for menopause:

- Brown rice provides complex carbohydrates, fiber, and B vitamins, which can help maintain energy levels and support overall health during menopause.

- Avocado is a great source of healthy fats, fiber, and antioxidants, which can help reduce inflammation and support cardiovascular health.

These colorful and nutritious vegan sushi rolls are a delicious and satisfying meal or snack that can support overall well•being during menopause, providing a balance of complex carbohydrates, healthy fats, and fiber•rich vegetables.

29. Greek Salad with Tofu Feta

Ingredient:

Tofu Feta:
- 1 block (14 oz) extra•firm tofu, drained and pressed
- 2 tbsp lemon juice
- 1 tbsp apple cider vinegar
- 1 tsp dried oregano
- 1/2 tsp garlic powder
- 1/4 tsp salt

Salad:
- 1 head romaine lettuce, chopped
- 1 cup cherry tomatoes, halved
- 1 cucumber, diced
- 1/2 red onion, thinly sliced
- 1/2 cup kalamata olives, pitted and halved
- 1/4 cup fresh parsley, chopped
- 2 tbsp extra•virgin olive oil
- 1 tbsp red wine vinegar
- 1 tsp dried oregano
- Salt and pepper to taste

Instructions:

Tofu Feta:

1. Cut the pressed tofu into 1/2•inch cubes and place in a shallow dish.
2. In a small bowl, whisk together the lemon juice, apple cider vinegar, dried oregano, garlic powder, and salt.
3. Pour the marinade over the tofu cubes and gently toss to coat. Cover and refrigerate for at least 30 minutes (or up to 24 hours).

Salad:

1. In a large salad bowl, combine the chopped romaine lettuce, cherry tomatoes, diced cucumber, sliced red onion, kalamata olives, and chopped parsley.
2. In a small bowl, whisk together the olive oil, red wine vinegar, and dried oregano. Season with salt and pepper to taste.
3. Add the marinated tofu feta to the salad and drizzle the dressing over the top. Gently toss to combine.

This vegan Greek salad is packed with nutrient•dense ingredients that can help support women during menopause, such as leafy greens, vegetables, healthy fats, and plant•based protein from the tofu feta.

30. Mushroom and Barley Soup

Ingredient:

- 1 tbsp olive oil
- 1 onion, diced
- 3 cloves garlic, minced
- 8 oz cremini or button mushrooms, sliced
- 4 cups low•sodium vegetable broth
- 1 cup pearl barley, rinsed
- 2 carrots, peeled and diced
- 2 celery stalks, diced
- 1 tsp dried thyme
- 1 tsp dried rosemary
- Salt and pepper to taste
- Chopped fresh parsley for garnish (optional)

Instructions:

1. In a large pot or Dutch oven, heat the olive oil over medium heat. Add the diced onion and minced garlic. Sauté for 2•3 minutes until fragrant.

2. Add the sliced mushrooms to the pot and cook for 5•7 minutes, stirring occasionally, until the mushrooms are tender and lightly browned.

3. Pour in the vegetable broth and add the rinsed pearl barley, diced carrots, and diced celery. Stir in the dried thyme and rosemary.

4. Bring the soup to a boil, then reduce the heat to low. Simmer for 30•40 minutes, or until the barley is tender.

5. Season the soup with salt and pepper to taste.

6. Ladle the mushroom and barley soup into bowls and garnish with chopped fresh parsley, if desired.

This vegan mushroom and barley soup is a nourishing and comforting meal that can be beneficial for women during menopause. The barley provides soluble fiber, which can help regulate digestion, while the mushrooms and vegetables offer a variety of vitamins, minerals, and antioxidants.

The earthy, savory flavors of this soup make it a satisfying and warming dish, perfect for a cozy meal. Enjoy!

31. Stir•fried Vegetables with Tempeh

Ingredient:

* 8 oz tempeh, cut into 1•inch cubes
* 2 tbsp low•sodium soy sauce or tamari
* 1 tbsp rice vinegar
* 1 tsp sesame oil
* 2 tbsp olive oil
* 3 cloves garlic, minced
* 1 inch fresh ginger, grated
* 1 red bell pepper, sliced
* 1 cup broccoli florets
* 1 cup sliced mushrooms
* 1 cup shredded cabbage
* 2 cups baby spinach
* 2 tbsp toasted sesame seeds
* Salt and pepper to taste

Instructions:

1. In a small bowl, combine the soy sauce/tamari, rice vinegar, and sesame oil. Set aside.

2. Heat the olive oil in a large skillet or wok over medium•high heat. Add the tempeh cubes and cook for 3•4 minutes per side until lightly browned. Transfer to a plate.

3. In the same skillet, add the garlic and ginger. Cook for 1 minute until fragrant.

4. Add the sliced bell pepper, broccoli, mushrooms, and cabbage. Stir•fry for 5•7 minutes until the vegetables are tender•crisp.

5. Add the spinach and the soy sauce mixture. Toss everything together until the spinach is wilted, about 2 minutes.

6. Return the cooked tempeh to the skillet and gently mix everything together.

7. Sprinkle the toasted sesame seeds over the top.

8. Season with salt and pepper to taste.

Serve the stir•fried vegetables and tempeh over brown rice or quinoa for a complete, nutrient•dense meal. The tempeh provides plant•based protein, while the vegetables offer fiber, vitamins, and minerals that can help support women during menopause.

32. Spaghetti Squash with Marinara Sauce

Ingredient:

- 1 medium spaghetti squash (about 3 lbs)
- 2 tbsp olive oil
- Salt and pepper to taste
- 1 (28 oz) can crushed tomatoes
- 2 cloves garlic, minced
- 1 tsp dried basil
- 1 tsp dried oregano
- 1/4 tsp red pepper flakes (optional)
- Freshly grated Parmesan cheese (optional)
- Chopped fresh basil for garnish (optional)

Instructions:

1. Preheat your oven to 400°F (200°C).

2. Cut the spaghetti squash in half lengthwise and scoop out the seeds. Brush the cut sides with 1 tbsp of the olive oil and season with salt and pepper.

3. Place the spaghetti squash halves cut•side down on a baking sheet. Roast for 40•50 minutes, or until the squash is tender and easily shreds with a fork.

4. While the spaghetti squash is roasting, prepare the marinara sauce. In a medium saucepan, heat the remaining 1 tbsp of olive oil over medium heat. Add the minced garlic and sauté for 1 minute until fragrant.

5. Pour in the crushed tomatoes and stir in the dried basil, dried oregano, and red pepper flakes (if using). Season with salt and pepper to taste.

6. Bring the marinara sauce to a simmer and let it cook for 10•15 minutes, stirring occasionally, to allow the flavors to meld.

7. Once the spaghetti squash is cooked, use a fork to shred the flesh into spaghetti•like strands.

8. Divide the spaghetti squash strands among plates or bowls. Top with the warm marinara sauce. If desired, garnish with freshly grated Parmesan cheese and chopped fresh basil.

33. Vegan Chili with Beans and Quinoa

Ingredient:

- 1 tbsp olive oil
- 1 onion, diced
- 3 cloves garlic, minced
- 1 red bell pepper, diced
- 2 carrots, peeled and diced
- 2 celery stalks, diced
- 1 jalapeño, seeded and minced (optional, for spice)
- 2 (15 oz) cans diced tomatoes
- 1 (15 oz) can black beans, drained and rinsed
- 1 (15 oz) can kidney beans, drained and rinsed
- 1 cup cooked quinoa
- 2 tbsp chili powder
- 1 tsp ground cumin
- 1 tsp dried oregano
- 1 tsp smoked paprika
- Salt and pepper to taste
- Chopped cilantro for garnish (optional)

Instructions:

1. In a large pot or Dutch oven, heat the olive oil over medium heat. Add the diced onion and minced garlic. Sauté for 2•3 minutes until fragrant.

2. Add the diced bell pepper, carrots, celery, and jalapeño (if using). Cook for 5•7 minutes, stirring occasionally, until the vegetables are tender.

3. Pour in the diced tomatoes, black beans, and kidney beans. Stir to combine.

4. Add the cooked quinoa, chili powder, cumin, oregano, and smoked paprika. Season with salt and pepper to taste.

5. Bring the chili to a simmer and let it cook for 15•20 minutes, stirring occasionally, to allow the flavors to meld. Taste and adjust seasonings as needed. Serve the vegan chili hot, garnished with chopped cilantro if desired.

This hearty vegan chili is packed with plant•based protein from the beans and quinoa, as well as fiber, vitamins, and minerals from the vegetables. It's a comforting and nutritious meal that can be enjoyed on its own or served with cornbread, tortilla chips, or a fresh salad.

34. Eggplant Parmesan

Ingredient:

- 2 medium eggplants, sliced into 1/2•inch thick rounds
- 1 cup all•purpose flour
- 2 eggs, beaten
- 2 cups panko breadcrumbs
- 1/2 cup grated Parmesan cheese
- 2 tbsp olive oil, plus more for frying
- 1 (24 oz) jar marinara sauce
- 8 oz shredded mozzarella cheese

Instructions:

1. Preheat your oven to 375°F (190°C).

2. Set up a breading station with three shallow dishes: one with the flour, one with the beaten eggs, and one with the panko breadcrumbs mixed with the Parmesan cheese.

3. Dredge the eggplant slices in the flour, dip them in the egg, and then coat them in the breadcrumb mixture, pressing gently to adhere.

4. In a large skillet, heat about 1/4 inch of olive oil over medium•high heat. Working in batches, fry the breaded eggplant slices for 2•3 minutes per side, or until golden brown. Transfer the fried eggplant slices to a paper towel•lined plate.

5. In a 9x13 inch baking dish, spread a thin layer of marinara sauce on the bottom. Arrange a single layer of the fried eggplant slices on top of the sauce.

6. Top the eggplant layer with more marinara sauce and sprinkle with some of the shredded mozzarella cheese.

7. Repeat the layers of eggplant, sauce, and mozzarella until all the ingredients are used up, ending with the mozzarella cheese on top.

8. Bake the eggplant Parmesan in the preheated oven for 25•30 minutes, or until the cheese is melted and bubbly. Let the dish cool for 5•10 minutes before serving.

Serve the eggplant Parmesan hot, garnished with fresh basil or parsley if desired. Enjoy this classic Italian•inspired dish!

35. Stuffed Portobello Mushrooms

Ingredient:

- 4 large portobello mushroom caps, stems removed and chopped
- 1 tbsp olive oil
- 1 onion, diced
- 3 cloves garlic, minced
- 1 cup cooked quinoa
- 1 (15 oz) can chickpeas, drained and rinsed
- 1/2 cup chopped spinach
- 2 tbsp chopped fresh basil
- 1 tsp dried oregano
- 1/4 cup unsweetened almond milk
- Salt and pepper to taste
- 1/4 cup shredded vegan mozzarella cheese (optional)

Instructions:

1. Preheat your oven to 400°F (200°C).

2. Gently clean the portobello mushroom caps with a damp cloth. Remove the stems and chop them.

3. In a large skillet, heat the olive oil over medium heat. Add the chopped mushroom stems, onion, and garlic. Sauté for 5•7 minutes until the vegetables are softened.

4. Stir in the cooked quinoa, drained and rinsed chickpeas, spinach, basil, and oregano. Cook for an additional 2•3 minutes, until the spinach is wilted.

5. Remove the skillet from heat and stir in the almond milk. Season with salt and pepper to taste.

6. Arrange the portobello mushroom caps, gill•side up, on a baking sheet. Spoon the quinoa and vegetable mixture evenly into the mushroom caps.

7. If using, sprinkle the shredded vegan mozzarella cheese over the top of the stuffed mushrooms.

8. Bake the stuffed mushrooms for 15•20 minutes, or until the mushrooms are tender and the filling is heated through.

9. Remove the stuffed mushrooms from the oven and let them cool for a few minutes before serving.

These vegan stuffed portobello mushrooms are a nutrient•dense and satisfying meal option for women during menopause. The quinoa, chickpeas, and spinach provide plant•based protein, fiber, and essential vitamins and minerals.

36. Sweet Potato and Black Bean Tacos

Ingredient:

- 2 medium sweet potatoes, peeled and diced
- 1 tbsp olive oil
- 1 tsp chili powder
- 1/2 tsp ground cumin
- Salt and pepper to taste
- 1 (15 oz) can black beans, drained and rinsed
- 1 cup diced red onion
- 2 cloves garlic, minced
- 1 jalapeño, seeded and minced (optional)
- 1 tsp lime juice
- 8•10 small corn or flour tortillas
- Toppings: shredded lettuce, diced avocado, salsa, cilantro, lime wedges

Instructions:

1. Preheat your oven to 400°F (200°C).

2. In a large bowl, toss the diced sweet potatoes with the olive oil, chili powder, cumin, and a pinch of salt and pepper.

3. Spread the seasoned sweet potato cubes in a single layer on a baking sheet. Roast for 20•25 minutes, stirring halfway, until the sweet potatoes are tender and lightly browned.

4. In a medium skillet, sauté the drained and rinsed black beans, diced red onion, minced garlic, and jalapeño (if using) over medium heat for 5•7 minutes, until the onions are translucent.

5. Remove the skillet from heat and stir in the lime juice. Season with salt and pepper to taste.

6. To assemble the tacos, divide the roasted sweet potatoes and black bean mixture evenly among the tortillas. Top the tacos with your desired toppings, such as shredded lettuce, diced avocado, salsa, cilantro, and a squeeze of lime juice.

Serve the sweet potato and black bean tacos immediately, while the sweet potatoes are still warm. These tacos make a delicious, nutritious, and easy•to•prepare meal. The combination of sweet potatoes, black beans, and fresh toppings creates a flavorful and satisfying taco experience.

37. Thai Peanut Noodles with Tofu

Ingredient:

- 8 oz whole wheat or brown rice noodles
- 1 block (14 oz) extra•firm tofu, pressed and cubed
- 2 tbsp sesame oil, divided
- 1 red bell pepper, sliced
- 2 cups shredded cabbage
- 1 cup shredded carrots
- 3 green onions, sliced
- 1/4 cup chopped fresh cilantro

Peanut Sauce:
- 1/2 cup creamy peanut butter
- 1/4 cup low•sodium soy sauce or tamari
- 2 tbsp rice vinegar
- 2 tbsp maple syrup
- 1 tbsp grated fresh ginger
- 1 clove garlic, minced
- 1/4 tsp red pepper flakes (optional)
- 1/4 cup unsweetened almond milk

Instructions:

1. Cook the noodles according to package instructions. Drain and rinse under cold water. Set aside.

2. In a large skillet or wok, heat 1 tbsp of the sesame oil over medium•high heat. Add the cubed tofu and sauté for 5•7 minutes, until lightly browned on all sides. Transfer the tofu to a plate.

3. In the same skillet, heat the remaining 1 tbsp of sesame oil. Add the sliced bell pepper, shredded cabbage, and shredded carrots. Sauté for 3•5 minutes, until the vegetables are tender•crisp.

4. In a medium bowl, whisk together all the peanut sauce ingredients until smooth and well combined.

5. Add the cooked noodles, sautéed vegetables, and tofu to the peanut sauce. Toss everything together until well coated.

6. Stir in the sliced green onions and chopped cilantro.

7. Serve the Thai peanut noodles warm, garnished with additional cilantro if desired.

This vegan Thai peanut noodle dish is packed with plant•based protein from the tofu, as well as fiber, vitamins, and minerals from the vegetables. The peanut sauce provides a creamy, flavorful coating that is both satisfying and nutritious.

The ingredients in this recipe can help support women during menopause by providing a balanced, nourishing meal.

38. Vegan Shepherd's Pie

Ingredient:

Filling:
- 1 tbsp olive oil
- 1 onion, diced
- 3 cloves garlic, minced
- 2 carrots, peeled and diced
- 2 celery stalks, diced
- 1 cup diced mushrooms
- 1 (15 oz) can lentils, drained and rinsed
- 1 (15 oz) can diced tomatoes
- 2 tbsp tomato paste

- 1 tsp dried thyme
- 1 tsp dried rosemary
- Salt and pepper to taste

Mashed Potato Topping:
- 3 lbs Yukon Gold potatoes, peeled and cubed
- 1/2 cup unsweetened almond milk
- 2 tbsp vegan butter or olive oil
- Salt and pepper to taste

Instructions:

1. Preheat your oven to 375°F (190°C).

2. In a large skillet, heat the olive oil over medium heat. Add the onion and garlic and sauté for 2•3 minutes until fragrant.

3. Add the carrots, celery, and mushrooms to the skillet. Cook for 5•7 minutes, stirring occasionally, until the vegetables are tender.

4. Stir in the drained and rinsed lentils, diced tomatoes, tomato paste, thyme, and rosemary. Season with salt and pepper to taste. Simmer for 10 minutes, allowing the flavors to meld.

5. Meanwhile, in a large pot, cover the cubed potatoes with water and bring to a boil. Reduce heat and simmer for 15•20 minutes, until the potatoes are tender. Drain the potatoes and return them to the pot.

6. Add the almond milk and vegan butter/olive oil to the potatoes. Mash until smooth and creamy. Season with salt and pepper to taste.

7. Transfer the lentil and vegetable filling to a 9x13 inch baking dish. Spread the mashed potatoes evenly over the top. Bake the shepherd's pie for 25•30 minutes, or until the potatoes are lightly browned on top. Remove from the oven and let cool for 5•10 minutes before serving.

This vegan shepherd's pie is packed with plant•based protein, fiber, and nutrients that can help support women during menopause. Enjoy!

39. Chickpea and Spinach Curry

Ingredient:

- 2 tbsp olive oil
- 1 onion, diced
- 3 cloves garlic, minced
- 1 tbsp grated fresh ginger
- 2 tsp garam masala
- 1 tsp ground cumin
- 1 tsp ground coriander
- 1/2 tsp ground turmeric
- 1/4 tsp cayenne pepper (or to taste)
- 1 (15 oz) can diced tomatoes
- 1 (15 oz) can chickpeas, drained and rinsed
- 1 (5 oz) bag baby spinach
- 1 cup coconut milk
- Salt and pepper to taste
- Chopped cilantro for garnish

Instructions:

1. In a large skillet or Dutch oven, heat the olive oil over medium heat. Add the diced onion and sauté for 3•4 minutes until translucent.

2. Add the minced garlic and grated ginger to the skillet. Cook for 1 minute, until fragrant.

3. Stir in the garam masala, cumin, coriander, turmeric, and cayenne pepper. Cook for 1•2 minutes to toast the spices.

4. Pour in the diced tomatoes and their juices. Bring the mixture to a simmer.

5. Add the drained and rinsed chickpeas to the skillet. Simmer for 5•7 minutes, allowing the flavors to meld.

6. Stir in the baby spinach and coconut milk. Cook for an additional 2•3 minutes, until the spinach is wilted.

7. Season the curry with salt and pepper to taste.

8. Serve the chickpea and spinach curry warm, garnished with chopped cilantro. Enjoy with basmati rice, naan bread, or your favorite accompaniments.

This flavorful curry is packed with plant•based protein from the chickpeas, as well as nutrient•dense spinach. The blend of aromatic spices and creamy coconut milk creates a delicious and comforting dish.

40. Grilled Vegetable Kebabs with Couscous

Ingredient:

Vegetable Kebabs:
- 1 red bell pepper, cut into 1•inch pieces
- 1 yellow bell pepper, cut into 1•inch pieces
- 1 zucchini, cut into 1•inch rounds
- 1 red onion, cut into 1•inch pieces
- 8 oz cremini mushrooms, halved
- 2 tbsp olive oil
- 1 tsp dried oregano
- Salt and pepper to taste

Couscous:
- 1 cup dry couscous
- 1 cup boiling water
- 1 tbsp olive oil
- 2 tbsp chopped fresh parsley
- 1 tbsp lemon juice
- Salt and pepper to taste

Instructions:

1. Preheat your grill or grill pan to medium•high heat.

2. In a large bowl, toss the cut vegetables with the olive oil, dried oregano, salt, and pepper until well coated.

3. Thread the seasoned vegetables onto skewers, leaving a little space between each piece.

4. Grill the vegetable kebabs for 12•15 minutes, turning occasionally, until the vegetables are tender and lightly charred.

5. While the kebabs are grilling, prepare the couscous. In a medium bowl, pour the boiling water over the dry couscous. Cover and let sit for 5 minutes.

6. Fluff the cooked couscous with a fork and stir in the olive oil, chopped parsley, lemon juice, salt, and pepper.

7. Serve the grilled vegetable kebabs warm, with the prepared couscous on the side.

Optional Additions:
- Sprinkle the couscous with toasted pine nuts or sliced almonds.
- Serve the kebabs and couscous with a dollop of hummus or tzatziki sauce.
- Add crumbled feta cheese to the couscous for extra flavor.

This grilled vegetable kebab and couscous dish is a delicious and healthy meal. The variety of colorful vegetables provide a range of vitamins, minerals, and antioxidants, while the couscous adds a satisfying base of complex carbohydrates.

41. Coconut Milk Ice Cream

Ingredient:

- 2 (13.5 oz) cans full•fat coconut milk
- 1/2 cup maple syrup
- 1 tsp vanilla extract
- 1/4 tsp sea salt
- 1/2 cup unsweetened shredded coconut (optional)

Instructions:

1. In a medium saucepan, whisk together the coconut milk, maple syrup, vanilla extract, and sea salt. Heat the mixture over medium heat, stirring occasionally, until it just begins to simmer.

2. Remove the saucepan from the heat and let the coconut milk mixture cool to room temperature.

3. Once cooled, transfer the mixture to a blender and blend until smooth and creamy.

4. Pour the blended coconut milk mixture into a shallow baking dish or a metal loaf pan. Cover and place in the freezer.

5. After 1 hour, remove the dish from the freezer and use a fork to stir and break up any frozen portions around the edges. This will help create a smooth, creamy texture.

6. Continue to freeze the ice cream, stirring every 30 minutes, for 2•3 hours, or until it reaches your desired consistency.

7. If using, stir in the unsweetened shredded coconut during the last 30 minutes of freezing.

8. Once the ice cream has reached your preferred texture, transfer it to an airtight container and freeze for at least 2 more hours before serving.

9. Scoop and serve the vegan coconut milk ice cream, garnished with additional shredded coconut if desired.

This dairy•free coconut milk ice cream is a delicious and nutritious treat that can be enjoyed by women during menopause. The healthy fats from the coconut milk, along with the natural sweetness of the maple syrup, make this a satisfying and menopause•friendly dessert.

42. Chia Seed Pudding with Mango

Ingredient:

- 1 cup unsweetened almond milk
- 1/4 cup chia seeds
- 2 tbsp maple syrup
- 1 tsp vanilla extract
- 1/2 tsp ground cinnamon
- 1 cup diced fresh mango
- 2 tbsp chopped pistachios (optional)

Instructions:

1. In a medium bowl, whisk together the almond milk, chia seeds, maple syrup, vanilla extract, and cinnamon until well combined.

2. Cover the bowl and refrigerate the chia seed pudding for at least 4 hours, or overnight, stirring occasionally, until thickened.

3. When ready to serve, divide the chia seed pudding evenly among 4 serving bowls or glasses.

4. Top each portion of chia pudding with 1/4 cup of diced fresh mango.

5. If desired, sprinkle the top of the pudding with the chopped pistachios for added crunch and texture.

6. Serve the chia seed pudding chilled.

This vegan chia seed pudding is a nutrient•dense and delicious breakfast or snack option that can be beneficial for women during menopause. The chia seeds provide fiber, protein, and omega•3 fatty acids, while the mango offers vitamins, minerals, and antioxidants.

The maple syrup provides a touch of natural sweetness, and the cinnamon may help regulate blood sugar levels. The optional pistachios add a satisfying crunch and healthy fats.

Enjoy this refreshing and menopause•friendly chia seed pudding with mango!

43. Vegan Chocolate Cake

Ingredient:

Cake:
* 2 cups all•purpose flour
* 2 cups granulated sugar
* 3/4 cup unsweetened cocoa powder
* 2 tsp baking soda
* 1 tsp baking powder
* 1 tsp salt
* 2 cups unsweetened almond milk
* 2/3 cup vegetable oil
* 2 tsp apple cider vinegar
* 2 tsp vanilla extract

Frosting:
* 1 cup vegan butter, softened
* 3 cups powdered sugar
* 1/3 cup unsweetened cocoa powder
* 1/4 cup unsweetened almond milk
* 1 tsp vanilla extract

Instructions:

1. Preheat your oven to 350°F (175°C). Grease and flour two 9•inch round cake pans.

2. In a large bowl, whisk together the flour, granulated sugar, cocoa powder, baking soda, baking powder, and salt.

3. In a separate bowl, combine the almond milk, vegetable oil, apple cider vinegar, and vanilla extract.

4. Pour the wet ingredients into the dry ingredients and whisk until just combined, being careful not to overmix. Divide the batter evenly between the prepared cake pans.

5. Bake for 30•35 minutes, or until a toothpick inserted into the center comes out clean. Allow the cakes to cool in the pans for 10 minutes, then transfer them to a wire rack to cool completely.

6. For the frosting, in a large bowl, beat the vegan butter with an electric mixer until light and fluffy. Gradually add the powdered sugar and cocoa powder, alternating with the almond milk, and beat until smooth and creamy.

7. Stir in the vanilla extract. Once the cakes are completely cooled, frost the top of one cake layer, then place the second layer on top. Frost the top and sides of the cake with the chocolate buttercream frosting. Refrigerate the cake for at least 2 hours before serving to allow the frosting to set.

This vegan chocolate cake is a decadent and menopause•friendly dessert. The almond milk and vegan butter provide healthy fats, while the cocoa powder and powdered sugar offer antioxidants and a touch of sweetness.

44. Baked Apples with Cinnamon

Ingredient:

- 4 medium•sized apples (such as Honeycrisp or Gala)
- 1/4 cup rolled oats
- 2 tbsp chopped walnuts
- 2 tbsp maple syrup
- 1 tsp ground cinnamon
- 1/4 tsp ground nutmeg
- 1/4 cup unsweetened almond milk (or other plant•based milk)

Instructions:

1. Preheat your oven to 375°F (190°C).

2. Wash the apples and use a sharp knife to cut off the top 1/4 of each apple. Scoop out the core and seeds, creating a small well in the center of each apple.

3. In a small bowl, mix together the rolled oats, chopped walnuts, maple syrup, cinnamon, and nutmeg.

4. Stuff the oat•nut mixture into the hollowed•out centers of the apples.

5. Place the stuffed apples in a baking dish and pour the almond milk around the base of the apples.

6. Bake for 30•35 minutes, or until the apples are tender and the filling is lightly browned.

7. Remove the baked apples from the oven and let them cool for a few minutes before serving.

Serve the baked apples warm, with the almond milk spooned over the top or on the side. The oats, walnuts, and cinnamon provide a delicious, comforting filling that is high in fiber, healthy fats, and antioxidants • all of which can be beneficial for women during menopause.

This dessert is naturally sweetened with maple syrup, making it a healthier alternative to traditional baked apple recipes. Enjoy!

45. Avocado Chocolate Mousse

Ingredient:

- 2 ripe avocados, pitted and flesh scooped out
- 1/2 cup unsweetened cocoa powder
- 1/2 cup maple syrup
- 1/4 cup unsweetened almond milk
- 1 tsp vanilla extract
- 1/4 tsp sea salt
- 1/4 cup chopped toasted walnuts (optional)

Instructions:

1. In a high•speed blender or food processor, combine the avocado flesh, cocoa powder, maple syrup, almond milk, vanilla extract, and sea salt. Blend until the mixture is smooth and creamy, scraping down the sides as needed.

2. Taste and adjust sweetness or other flavors as desired. The mousse should have a rich, chocolatey flavor.

3. Divide the avocado chocolate mousse evenly among 4•6 small serving dishes or ramekins.

4. Refrigerate the mousse for at least 2 hours, or until it has set and thickened to your desired consistency.

5. If using, sprinkle the chopped toasted walnuts over the top of the chilled mousse just before serving.

This vegan avocado chocolate mousse is a decadent and nutrient•dense dessert that can be enjoyed by women during menopause. The key benefits include:

- Avocados: Provide healthy fats, fiber, and antioxidants that can help support skin and heart health.
- Cocoa powder: Rich in flavonoids that may have anti•inflammatory properties.
- Maple syrup: A natural sweetener that provides trace minerals.
- Walnuts (optional): Offer omega•3 fatty acids, which can help reduce menopausal symptoms.

The creamy, rich texture of this mousse makes it a satisfying and indulgent treat that is also good for you. Enjoy this vegan avocado chocolate mousse as a delicious and menopause•friendly dessert.

46. Vegan Cheesecake with Berries

Ingredient:

Crust:
- 1 1/2 cups graham cracker crumbs (or crushed vegan cookies)
- 5 tbsp vegan butter, melted

Topping:
- 2 cups mixed fresh berries (such as raspberries, blueberries, and strawberries)
- 2 tbsp maple syrup (optional)

Filling:
- 1 cup raw cashews, soaked in water for at least 4 hours or overnight
- 1 (14 oz) can full•fat coconut milk
- 1/2 cup maple syrup
- 1/4 cup lemon juice
- 1 tsp vanilla extract
- 1/4 tsp sea salt

Instructions:

Crust:
1. Preheat your oven to 350°F (175°C). Grease a 9•inch springform pan.
2. In a medium bowl, mix together the graham cracker crumbs and melted vegan butter until well combined.
3. Press the crust mixture firmly into the bottom and up the sides of the prepared springform pan.
4. Bake the crust for 10 minutes, then let it cool completely.

Filling:
1. Drain and rinse the soaked cashews. Add them to a high•speed blender along with the coconut milk, maple syrup, lemon juice, vanilla, and salt.
2. Blend the mixture on high speed until completely smooth and creamy, about 2•3 minutes.
3. Pour the cheesecake filling into the cooled crust and smooth the top.
4. Refrigerate the cheesecake for at least 4 hours, or until set.

Topping:
1. When ready to serve, arrange the fresh berries on top of the chilled cheesecake.
2. If desired, drizzle the berries with a bit of maple syrup.

Slice and serve the vegan cheesecake with berries. Store any leftovers in the refrigerator.

This vegan cheesecake is a delicious and indulgent dessert that is also nutritious. The cashews provide a creamy texture, while the coconut milk and maple syrup add richness and sweetness. The fresh berries on top provide a vibrant, flavorful contrast.

47. Banana Nice Cream

Ingredient:

- 4 ripe bananas, peeled and frozen
- 1/2 cup unsweetened almond milk
- 2 tbsp almond butter
- 1 tsp vanilla extract
- 1/4 tsp ground cinnamon
- Pinch of sea salt

Optional Toppings:
- Chopped nuts (such as almonds or walnuts)
- Fresh berries (such as strawberries or blueberries)
- Unsweetened shredded coconut
- Drizzle of maple syrup or honey

Instructions:

1. In a high•speed blender or food processor, combine the frozen banana slices, almond milk, almond butter, vanilla extract, cinnamon, and sea salt.

2. Blend the ingredients on high speed, stopping to scrape down the sides as needed, until the mixture is smooth and creamy, resembling soft•serve ice cream.

3. Scoop the banana nice cream into bowls or cups.

4. Top the nice cream with your desired toppings, such as chopped nuts, fresh berries, shredded coconut, or a drizzle of maple syrup or honey. Serve immediately, or transfer the nice cream to an airtight container and freeze for 1•2 hours for a firmer texture.

This vegan banana nice cream is a delicious and nutritious treat that can be enjoyed by women during menopause. The key ingredients provide the following benefits:
- Bananas: Rich in potassium, which can help regulate blood pressure and reduce the risk of heart disease.

- Almond milk: Provides calcium and other minerals that are important for bone health.

- Almond butter: Contains healthy fats, protein, and magnesium, which can help manage menopausal symptoms.

- Cinnamon: May have anti•inflammatory properties and help regulate blood sugar levels.

48. Almond Flour Cookies

Ingredient:

- 2 cups almond flour
- 1/4 cup coconut flour
- 1/4 cup maple syrup
- 1/4 cup coconut oil, melted
- 1 tsp vanilla extract
- 1/4 tsp sea salt
- 1/2 cup chopped walnuts (optional)

Instructions:

1. Preheat your oven to 350°F (175°C). Line a baking sheet with parchment paper.

2. In a large bowl, whisk together the almond flour and coconut flour.

3. Add the maple syrup, melted coconut oil, vanilla extract, and sea salt. Stir until a dough forms.

4. If using, fold in the chopped walnuts.

5. Scoop the dough by the tablespoonful and place the cookies about 2 inches apart on the prepared baking sheet. Gently flatten each cookie with the back of a fork.

6. Bake the cookies for 12•15 minutes, or until lightly golden around the edges. Remove the cookies from the oven and let them cool on the baking sheet for 5 minutes before transferring them to a wire rack to cool completely.

These vegan almond flour cookies are a delicious and nutritious treat that can be enjoyed by women during menopause. The key benefits include:

- Almond flour: Provides healthy fats, protein, and fiber to help support overall health.

- Coconut flour: Rich in fiber, which can help regulate digestion.

- Maple syrup: A natural sweetener that contains antioxidants and minerals.

- Coconut oil: Contains medium•chain triglycerides (MCTs) that may have beneficial effects on brain and metabolic health. Offer omega•3 fatty acids, which can help reduce inflammation.

49. Raspberry Chia Jam Bars

Ingredient:

Crust and Topping:
- 1 1/2 cups rolled oats
- 1 cup whole wheat flour
- 1/2 cup unsweetened shredded coconut
- 1/2 cup packed brown sugar
- 1/2 tsp baking soda
- 1/4 tsp salt
- 1/2 cup unsalted butter, melted

Chia Jam Filling:
- 2 cups fresh or frozen raspberries
- 2 tbsp chia seeds
- 2 tbsp maple syrup
- 1 tsp vanilla extract

Instructions:

1. Preheat your oven to 350°F (175°C). Grease an 8x8 inch baking pan.

Crust and Topping:

2. In a large bowl, combine the rolled oats, whole wheat flour, shredded coconut, brown sugar, baking soda, and salt. Mix well.
3. Pour in the melted butter and stir until the mixture is well combined and crumbly.
4. Set aside 1 cup of the oat mixture for the topping.
5. Press the remaining oat mixture evenly into the bottom of the prepared baking pan.

Chia Jam Filling:

6. In a medium saucepan, combine the raspberries, chia seeds, maple syrup, and vanilla extract. Cook over medium heat, stirring frequently, until the mixture thickens, about 5•7 minutes.
7. Spread the chia jam evenly over the crust in the baking pan.
8. Sprinkle the reserved 1 cup of oat mixture over the top of the jam.

9. Bake for 25•30 minutes, or until the top is lightly golden.
10. Allow the bars to cool completely in the pan before cutting into squares.

Serve the raspberry chia jam bars at room temperature or chilled. They make a delicious and nutritious snack or dessert.

50. Carrot Cake with Cashew Frosting

Ingredient:

Carrot Cake:
- 2 cups all•purpose flour
- 2 teaspoons baking powder
- 1 teaspoon baking soda
- 1 teaspoon ground cinnamon
- 1/4 teaspoon ground nutmeg
- 1/4 teaspoon salt
- 3 large eggs
- 1 1/4 cups granulated sugar
- 3/4 cup vegetable or canola oil
- 1 teaspoon vanilla extract
- 3 cups grated carrots (about 6•8 medium carrots)

Cashew Frosting:
- 1 cup raw cashews, soaked in water for at least 4 hours or overnight
- 1/2 cup unsweetened almond milk
- 1/4 cup maple syrup
- 1 teaspoon vanilla extract
- 1/4 teaspoon salt

Instructions:

1. Preheat oven to 350°F. Grease a 9x13 inch baking pan.

2. In a medium bowl, whisk together the flour, baking powder, baking soda, cinnamon, nutmeg and salt.

3. In a large bowl, beat the eggs and sugar together until light and fluffy. Slowly pour in the oil and vanilla and mix until combined.

4. Fold in the grated carrots.

5. Gradually mix the dry ingredients into the wet ingredients until just combined.

6. Pour the batter into the prepared baking pan and bake for 30•35 minutes, until a toothpick inserted in the center comes out clean.

7. Allow the cake to cool completely.

8. For the frosting, drain and rinse the soaked cashews. Add them to a high•speed blender or food processor along with the almond milk, maple syrup, vanilla and salt. Blend until completely smooth and creamy.

9. Spread the cashew frosting evenly over the top of the cooled cake. Refrigerate the cake for at least 2 hours before serving to allow the frosting to set.

51. Green Tea Smoothie

Ingredient:

- 1 cup unsweetened almond milk
- 1 cup packed baby spinach
- 1 ripe banana, frozen
- 1 tbsp matcha green tea powder
- 1 tbsp almond butter
- 1 tsp honey or maple syrup (optional)
- 1/2 tsp ground ginger
- 1/4 tsp ground turmeric
- Ice cubes (optional)

Instructions:

1. In a high•speed blender, combine the unsweetened almond milk, baby spinach, frozen banana, matcha green tea powder, almond butter, honey/maple syrup (if using), ground ginger, and ground turmeric.

2. Blend the ingredients on high speed until the mixture is smooth and creamy, about 1•2 minutes.

3. If you'd like a thicker, colder smoothie, add a few ice cubes and blend again until the desired consistency is reached.

4. Pour the green tea smoothie into a glass and enjoy immediately.

This vegan green tea smoothie is a nutrient•dense and refreshing beverage that can be beneficial for women during menopause. The key ingredients provide the following benefits:

- Spinach: Rich in vitamins, minerals, and antioxidants that can help support overall health.
- Matcha green tea: Contains L•theanine, which may help reduce stress and anxiety.
- Almond butter: Provides healthy fats, protein, and magnesium to help manage menopausal symptoms.
- Ginger and turmeric: Have anti•inflammatory properties that can help alleviate joint pain and other menopausal issues.

Feel free to adjust the sweetener (honey or maple syrup) to your personal taste preferences. You can also experiment with adding other nutrient•dense ingredients, such as chia seeds or flaxseeds, to boost the nutritional profile even further.

52. Turmeric Latte

Ingredient:

- 1 cup unsweetened almond milk or oat milk
- 1 tsp ground turmeric
- 1/2 tsp ground ginger
- 1/4 tsp ground cinnamon
- 1/8 tsp ground black pepper
- 1•2 tsp maple syrup or honey (optional)

Instructions:

1. In a small saucepan, whisk together the almond/oat milk, turmeric, ginger, cinnamon, and black pepper.

2. Heat the mixture over medium heat, whisking frequently, until steaming hot but not boiling.

3. Remove from heat and stir in 1•2 tsp of maple syrup or honey, if desired, to sweeten to taste. Pour the turmeric latte into a mug.

Why this recipe is tailored for menopause:

- Turmeric is a powerful anti•inflammatory spice that can help alleviate some of the common symptoms of menopause like joint pain, hot flashes, and mood swings.

- Ginger also has anti•inflammatory properties and can help settle the stomach, which can be helpful for menopausal women.

- Cinnamon may help regulate blood sugar levels, which can fluctuate during menopause.

- Black pepper enhances the bioavailability of turmeric, allowing your body to better absorb its beneficial compounds.

- Using plant•based milk like almond or oat milk makes this latte dairy•free, which can be easier on the digestive system during menopause. The optional maple syrup or honey provides a touch of sweetness without spiking blood sugar too much.

This comforting, nourishing turmeric latte is a great way for menopausal women to get an anti•inflammatory boost and some relief from common symptoms. Enjoy it as a soothing daily ritual.

53. Herbal Tea with Lemon Balm

Ingredient:

- 4 cups water
- 1/4 cup fresh lemon balm leaves
- 1 tbsp dried chamomile flowers (optional)
- 1 tbsp dried peppermint leaves (optional)
- 1•2 tbsp honey (optional)
- Lemon slices for garnish (optional)

Instructions:

1. In a medium saucepan, bring the water to a boil.

2. Remove the pan from heat and add the fresh lemon balm leaves. If using, also add the dried chamomile flowers and/or dried peppermint leaves.

3. Cover the saucepan and let the herbs steep for 5•7 minutes.

4. Strain the tea through a fine•mesh sieve to remove the herbs.

5. Pour the lemon balm tea into mugs.

6. If desired, stir in 1•2 tablespoons of honey to sweeten the tea.

7. Garnish each mug with a lemon slice.

Enjoy your soothing and fragrant herbal tea with lemon balm.

Lemon balm (Melissa officinalis) is an herb that has been used for centuries for its calming and relaxing properties. It is believed to have a positive effect on mood and can help alleviate stress and anxiety.

The addition of chamomile and peppermint further enhances the tea's soothing and restorative qualities, making it a great choice for women during menopause.

Feel free to adjust the amount of herbs to suit your personal taste preferences. This herbal tea can be enjoyed hot or chilled.

54. Matcha Latte with Almond Milk

Ingredient:

- 1 cup unsweetened almond milk
- 1 tsp matcha green tea powder
- 1•2 tsp maple syrup or honey (optional)
- 1/4 tsp ground cinnamon
- 1/8 tsp ground ginger

Instructions:

1. In a small saucepan, whisk together the almond milk, matcha powder, and maple syrup/honey (if using) until well combined.

2. Heat the mixture over medium heat, whisking frequently, until steaming hot but not boiling.

3. Remove from heat and stir in the ground cinnamon and ginger.

4. Pour the matcha latte into a mug and enjoy immediately.

Why this recipe is tailored for menopause:

• Matcha green tea is rich in antioxidants and L•theanine, which can help promote calm focus and reduce stress • both of which can be beneficial for menopausal women.

• Cinnamon may help regulate blood sugar levels, which can fluctuate during menopause.

• Ginger has anti•inflammatory properties that can help alleviate joint pain and other menopausal symptoms.

• Using unsweetened almond milk makes this latte dairy•free, which can be easier on the digestive system during menopause.

• The optional maple syrup or honey provides a touch of sweetness without spiking blood sugar too much.

This creamy, comforting matcha latte is a great way for menopausal women to get a boost of antioxidants and anti•inflammatory compounds, while also promoting a sense of calm. Enjoy it as a soothing daily ritual.

55. Chilled Hibiscus Tea

Ingredient:

- 6 cups water
- 1/2 cup dried hibiscus flowers (or 4•5 hibiscus tea bags)
- 2•3 tbsp honey or maple syrup (optional)
- 1 tsp ground ginger
- 1/2 tsp ground cinnamon
- Lemon or lime slices for serving (optional)

Instructions:

1. In a large saucepan, bring the water to a boil. Remove from heat and add the dried hibiscus flowers (or tea bags).

2. Allow the hibiscus to steep for 5•7 minutes, until the water has turned a deep red/pink color.

3. Strain the tea through a fine mesh sieve to remove the hibiscus flowers. Discard the flowers.

4. Stir in the honey or maple syrup (if using), ground ginger, and ground cinnamon until well combined.

5. Allow the tea to cool to room temperature, then refrigerate for at least 2 hours or until chilled. Serve the chilled hibiscus tea over ice, garnished with lemon or lime slices if desired.

Why this recipe is tailored for menopause:

- Hibiscus tea is rich in antioxidants and has been shown to help lower blood pressure, which can be beneficial for menopausal women.

- Ginger has anti•inflammatory properties that can help alleviate joint pain and other menopausal symptoms.

- Cinnamon may help regulate blood sugar levels, which can fluctuate during menopause.

This refreshing, chilled hibiscus tea is a great way for menopausal women to stay hydrated and get a boost of antioxidants and anti•inflammatory compounds. Enjoy it as a soothing daily ritual.

56. Ginger and Lemon Detox Drink

Ingredient:

- 4 cups filtered water
- 2 inches fresh ginger, peeled and sliced
- 2 lemons, juiced (about 1/4 cup lemon juice)
- 2 tbsp raw honey or maple syrup (optional)
- 1/4 tsp ground turmeric
- Pinch of black pepper

Instructions:

1. In a medium saucepan, bring the filtered water to a boil over high heat.

2. Add the sliced ginger and reduce the heat to medium•low. Simmer for 10•15 minutes to allow the ginger to infuse the water.

3. Remove the saucepan from the heat and stir in the lemon juice, honey/maple syrup (if using), turmeric, and black pepper.

4. Allow the mixture to cool slightly, then strain out the ginger slices.

5. Pour the detox drink into glasses and serve either warm or chilled over ice.

Why this recipe is tailored for menopause:

- Ginger is a powerful anti•inflammatory that can help alleviate joint pain, muscle aches, and other menopausal symptoms.

- Lemon is a good source of vitamin C, which can support the immune system during menopause.

- Turmeric is another potent anti•inflammatory that may help reduce hot flashes and mood swings.

- Black pepper enhances the bioavailability of turmeric, allowing your body to better absorb its beneficial compounds.

This refreshing, ginger•lemon detox drink is a great way for menopausal women to get a boost of anti•inflammatory nutrients and support their body's natural detoxification processes. Enjoy it daily as part of a healthy lifestyle.

57. Almond Milk Hot Chocolate

Ingredient:

- 2 cups unsweetened almond milk
- 2 tbsp unsweetened cocoa powder
- 1 tbsp maple syrup or honey
- 1/2 tsp ground cinnamon
- 1/4 tsp ground ginger
- 1/8 tsp ground nutmeg
- Pinch of sea salt

Optional Toppings:
- Whipped coconut cream
- Chopped toasted almonds
- Shaved dark chocolate

Instructions:

1. In a small saucepan, whisk together the almond milk, cocoa powder, maple syrup/honey, cinnamon, ginger, nutmeg, and salt.

2. Heat the mixture over medium heat, whisking frequently, until steaming hot and well combined, about 5 minutes. Do not boil.

3. Remove from heat and pour the hot chocolate into mugs. Top with whipped coconut cream, chopped toasted almonds, and/or shaved dark chocolate, if desired.

Why this recipe is tailored for menopause:

- Almond milk is dairy•free, which can be easier on the digestive system during menopause.

- Cinnamon may help regulate blood sugar levels, which can fluctuate during menopause.

- Ginger has anti•inflammatory properties that can help alleviate joint pain and other menopausal symptoms.

- Nutmeg contains compounds that may help reduce anxiety and improve sleep, both of which can be issues for menopausal women.

This rich, creamy hot chocolate is a comforting and nourishing treat that can provide some relief from common menopausal symptoms. Enjoy it as a soothing daily ritual.

58. Beetroot Smoothie

Ingredient:

- 1 cup unsweetened almond milk
- 1 cup frozen cubed beets
- 1 frozen banana
- 1 tbsp ground flaxseed
- 1 tbsp almond butter
- 1 tsp ground cinnamon
- 1/2 tsp ground ginger
- 1/4 tsp ground turmeric
- Pinch of black pepper

Instructions:

1. Add all the ingredients to a high•speed blender and blend until smooth and creamy.

2. Pour the smoothie into a glass and enjoy immediately.

Why this recipe is tailored for menopause:

• Beets are a great source of folate, which can help support healthy hormone levels during menopause.

• The antioxidants in beets may help reduce inflammation and alleviate some menopausal symptoms like hot flashes.

• Cinnamon can help regulate blood sugar levels, which can fluctuate during menopause.

• Ginger has anti•inflammatory properties that can help with joint pain and other menopausal symptoms.

• Turmeric is a powerful anti•inflammatory spice that can also help with mood and cognitive function.

• Flaxseed is a great source of plant•based omega•3 fatty acids, which can help support brain and heart health during menopause.

This vibrant, nutrient•dense smoothie is a great way for menopausal women to get a boost of antioxidants, anti•inflammatory compounds, and essential nutrients to help alleviate common symptoms. Enjoy it as a refreshing and nourishing breakfast or snack.

59. Chia Fresca with Lime

Ingredient:

- 4 cups filtered water
- 2 tbsp chia seeds
- 2 tbsp freshly squeezed lime juice (about 1 lime)
- 1•2 tbsp maple syrup or honey (optional)
- Pinch of sea salt

Instructions:

1. In a large pitcher or jar, combine the filtered water and chia seeds. Stir well and let sit for 10•15 minutes, stirring occasionally, until the chia seeds have formed a gel•like consistency.

2. Add the freshly squeezed lime juice, maple syrup/honey (if using), and a pinch of sea salt. Stir to combine.

3. Taste and adjust sweetener as needed. The lime juice and chia seeds provide natural sweetness, so you may not need much additional sweetener. Serve the chia fresca over ice. Garnish with extra lime slices if desired.

Why this recipe is tailored for menopause:

- Chia seeds are a great source of omega•3 fatty acids, which can help reduce inflammation and support brain health during menopause.

- Lime is rich in vitamin C, which can help boost the immune system and support collagen production, important for skin health during menopause.

- The optional maple syrup or honey provides a touch of sweetness without spiking blood sugar too much, which can be helpful for menopausal women.

- Staying hydrated is crucial during menopause, and the chia seeds in this drink help provide a boost of fiber and nutrients.

- The refreshing, slightly tart flavor of this chia fresca can be a nice alternative to sugary drinks for menopausal women.

This simple, nourishing chia fresca is a great way for menopausal women to stay hydrated, get a boost of anti•inflammatory nutrients, and support their overall health. Enjoy it as a refreshing daily beverage.

60. Golden Milk with Coconut Milk

Ingredient:

- 1 cup unsweetened coconut milk
- 1 cup unsweetened almond milk
- 1 tbsp ground turmeric
- 1 tsp ground ginger
- 1/2 tsp ground cinnamon
- 1/4 tsp ground black pepper
- 1•2 tsp maple syrup or honey (optional)

Instructions:

1. In a small saucepan, whisk together the coconut milk, almond milk, turmeric, ginger, cinnamon, and black pepper.

2. Heat the mixture over medium heat, whisking frequently, until steaming hot but not boiling.

3. Remove from heat and stir in 1•2 tsp of maple syrup or honey, if desired, to sweeten to taste. Pour the golden milk into mugs and enjoy immediately.

Why this recipe is tailored for menopause:

- Turmeric is a powerful anti•inflammatory spice that can help alleviate joint pain, hot flashes, and mood swings associated with menopause.

- Ginger also has anti•inflammatory properties and can help settle the stomach, which can be beneficial for menopausal women.

- Cinnamon may help regulate blood sugar levels, which can fluctuate during menopause.

- Black pepper enhances the bioavailability of turmeric, allowing your body to better absorb its beneficial compounds.

- Coconut milk is a rich source of healthy fats that can support skin, hair, and hormone health during menopause.

This comforting, nourishing golden milk is a great way for menopausal women to get an anti•inflammatory boost and some relief from common symptoms. Enjoy it as a soothing daily ritual.

61. Stuffed Avocados with Black Beans

Ingredient:

- 4 ripe avocados, halved and pits removed
- 1 (15 oz) can black beans, rinsed and drained
- 1/2 cup diced red onion
- 1/2 cup diced tomatoes
- 2 tbsp chopped fresh cilantro
- 2 tbsp freshly squeezed lime juice
- 1 tsp ground cumin
- 1/2 tsp chili powder
- 1/4 tsp garlic powder
- Salt and pepper to taste

Instructions:

1. In a medium bowl, combine the black beans, red onion, tomatoes, cilantro, lime juice, cumin, chili powder, and garlic powder. Season with salt and pepper to taste.

2. Scoop the black bean mixture evenly into the avocado halves.

3. Serve the stuffed avocados immediately, or refrigerate until ready to serve.

Why this recipe is tailored for menopause:

- Avocados are a great source of healthy fats, which can help support skin, hair, and hormone health during menopause.

- Black beans are high in fiber, which can help regulate digestion and blood sugar levels.

- Onions and tomatoes are rich in antioxidants that can help reduce inflammation.

- Cilantro is a cooling herb that may help alleviate hot flashes and night sweats.

- Lime juice provides a boost of vitamin C, which supports the immune system.

- Cumin, chili powder, and garlic have anti•inflammatory properties that can help with joint pain and other menopausal symptoms.

This stuffed avocado dish is a nutrient•dense, flavorful, and satisfying option for menopausal women. The combination of healthy fats, fiber, and anti•inflammatory ingredients can help provide relief from common menopausal symptoms.

62. Vegan Spinach Artichoke Dip

Ingredient:

- 1 cup raw cashews, soaked in water for at least 4 hours or overnight
- 1 (14 oz) can artichoke hearts, drained and chopped
- 1 (10 oz) package frozen chopped spinach, thawed and drained
- 1/2 cup unsweetened almond milk
- 2 tbsp fresh lemon juice
- 2 tsp Dijon mustard
- 1 tsp garlic powder
- 1/2 tsp onion powder
- 1/2 tsp dried thyme
- 1/4 tsp ground nutmeg
- Salt and pepper to taste

Serving suggestions:
- Whole grain crackers or sliced vegetables (such as carrots, celery, cucumber)

Instructions:

1. Drain and rinse the soaked cashews. Add them to a high•speed blender or food processor along with the almond milk, lemon juice, Dijon mustard, garlic powder, onion powder, thyme, and nutmeg. Blend until smooth and creamy.

2. In a medium bowl, mix the blended cashew mixture with the chopped artichoke hearts and spinach. Season with salt and pepper to taste.

3. Transfer the spinach artichoke dip to a serving bowl. Serve immediately with whole grain crackers or sliced vegetables.

Why this recipe is tailored for menopause:

• Cashews provide a creamy, protein•rich base without any dairy. Spinach is a great source of folate, which can help support healthy hormone levels during menopause.

• Artichokes are high in fiber and antioxidants, which can help reduce inflammation. Lemon juice provides a boost of vitamin C to support the immune system.

• Garlic, onion, and thyme have anti•inflammatory properties that can help with joint pain and other menopausal symptoms. Nutmeg contains compounds that may help improve mood and sleep.

63. Mini Cucumber Sandwiches

Ingredient:

- 1 English cucumber, sliced into 1/4•inch rounds
- 1 cup vegan cream cheese (such as Kite Hill or Treeline)
- 2 tbsp chopped fresh dill
- 1 tbsp lemon juice
- 1/4 tsp garlic powder
- 1/4 tsp ground black pepper
- Pinch of sea salt
- 8•10 slices whole grain or gluten•free bread, crusts removed and cut into quarters

Instructions:

1. In a small bowl, mix together the vegan cream cheese, dill, lemon juice, garlic powder, black pepper, and salt until well combined.

2. Spread a thin layer of the cream cheese mixture onto each bread quarter.

3. Top each bread quarter with a slice of cucumber.

4. Arrange the mini cucumber sandwiches on a serving platter. Refrigerate for at least 30 minutes before serving to allow the flavors to meld.

Why this recipe is tailored for menopause:

- Cucumbers are hydrating and contain silica, which supports skin and bone health during menopause.

- Dill is a cooling herb that may help alleviate hot flashes and night sweats.

- Lemon juice provides a boost of vitamin C, which can support the immune system.

- Garlic has anti•inflammatory properties that can help with joint pain.

- The vegan cream cheese provides a creamy, protein•rich base without any dairy. Whole grain or gluten•free bread options are gentler on the digestive system.

These mini cucumber sandwiches make for a refreshing, nourishing, and easy•to•prepare snack or appetizer for menopausal women. The combination of cooling, anti•inflammatory, and immune•boosting ingredients can help provide relief from common menopausal symptoms.

64. Cauliflower Buffalo Wings

Ingredient:

- 1 head of cauliflower, cut into bite•sized florets
- 1 cup all•purpose flour
- 1 cup unsweetened almond milk (or regular milk)
- 1 tsp garlic powder
- 1 tsp onion powder
- 1/2 tsp salt
- 1/4 tsp black pepper
- 1/2 cup hot sauce (such as Frank's RedHot)
- 2 tbsp melted butter or vegan butter

Instructions:

1. Preheat oven to 450°F. Line a baking sheet with parchment paper.

2. In a large bowl, whisk together the flour, almond milk, garlic powder, onion powder, salt, and pepper until a smooth batter forms.

3. Add the cauliflower florets to the batter and toss to coat evenly.

4. Arrange the battered cauliflower in a single layer on the prepared baking sheet.

5. Bake for 20•25 minutes, flipping halfway, until the cauliflower is golden brown and crispy.

6. In a small bowl, whisk together the hot sauce and melted butter.

7. Toss the baked cauliflower with the buffalo sauce until evenly coated.

8. Serve immediately, with ranch or blue cheese dressing for dipping if desired. Enjoy!

65. Gazpacho Soup

Ingredient:

- 4 large tomatoes, chopped
- 1 cucumber, peeled, seeded and chopped
- 1 red bell pepper, chopped
- 1 small red onion, chopped
- 2 garlic cloves, minced
- 2 cups tomato juice
- 2 tbsp red wine vinegar
- 1 tbsp olive oil
- 1 tsp Worcestershire sauce
- 1 tsp Tabasco sauce
- 1 tsp salt
- 1/4 tsp black pepper
- Chopped fresh parsley, for garnish

Instructions:

1. In a large bowl, combine the chopped tomatoes, cucumber, bell pepper, onion and garlic.

2. Add the tomato juice, red wine vinegar, olive oil, Worcestershire sauce, Tabasco, salt and pepper. Stir to combine.

3. Cover and refrigerate for at least 2 hours, or up to 24 hours, to allow the flavors to meld.

4. When ready to serve, give the gazpacho a good stir. Ladle into bowls and garnish with chopped fresh parsley.

5. Serve chilled, with crusty bread on the side if desired.

Tips:
- For a smoother texture, you can blend part of the gazpacho in a food processor or blender before stirring it back into the chunky vegetables.
- Add diced avocado, croutons or a dollop of sour cream as optional toppings.
- Adjust seasoning to taste, adding more vinegar, Tabasco or salt as needed.

Enjoy this refreshing, no•cook Spanish•style cold tomato soup!

66. Vegan Spring Rolls with Peanut Sauce

Ingredient:

- 8•10 rice paper wrappers
- 2 cups shredded cabbage
- 1 cup shredded carrots
- 1 cup thinly sliced cucumber
- 1 cup cooked and cooled brown rice vermicelli noodles
- 1/2 cup fresh mint leaves
- 1/2 cup fresh cilantro leaves

Peanut Sauce Ingredients:
- 1/2 cup creamy peanut butter
- 1/4 cup unsweetened almond milk
- 2 tbsp low•sodium soy sauce or tamari
- 1 tbsp rice vinegar
- 1 tbsp maple syrup
- 1 tsp sesame oil
- 1 tsp grated fresh ginger
- 1/4 tsp ground turmeric
- Pinch of cayenne pepper (optional)

Instructions:

1. Make the peanut sauce by blending all the sauce ingredients together until smooth. Set aside.

2. Fill a shallow bowl with warm water. Dip one rice paper wrapper into the water for 10•15 seconds until softened.

3. Place the softened wrapper on a clean, damp surface. Layer a small amount of the cabbage, carrots, cucumber, noodles, mint, and cilantro in the center.

4. Fold the bottom of the wrapper up over the filling, then fold in the sides and continue rolling tightly into a cylinder.

5. Repeat with the remaining wrappers and fillings. Serve the spring rolls immediately with the peanut sauce for dipping.

This fresh, veggie•packed spring roll dish is a delicious and nourishing option for menopausal women. Enjoy it as a light meal or appetizer.

67. Zucchini Fritters

Ingredient:

- 3 medium zucchini, grated (about 3 cups)
- 1/2 cup all•purpose flour (or gluten•free flour)
- 1/4 cup unsweetened almond milk
- 2 tbsp ground flaxseed
- 1 tsp baking powder
- 1/2 tsp salt
- 1/4 tsp black pepper
- 2 tbsp olive oil, plus more for cooking

For the Lemon Dill Sauce:

- 1/2 cup unsweetened vegan yogurt (such as almond or coconut)
- 1 tbsp lemon juice
- 1 tbsp chopped fresh dill
- 1/4 tsp salt

Instructions:

1. Grate the zucchini using a box grater or food processor. Place the grated zucchini in a clean kitchen towel or cheesecloth and squeeze out as much moisture as possible.

2. In a medium bowl, whisk together the flour, almond milk, ground flaxseed, baking powder, salt and pepper until a thick batter forms. Fold in the grated zucchini.

3. In a large skillet, heat 1•2 tbsp of olive oil over medium heat. Scoop heaping tablespoons of the zucchini batter into the hot oil, flattening them slightly.

4. Cook the fritters for 2•3 minutes per side, until golden brown. Transfer to a paper towel•lined plate.

5. Repeat with the remaining zucchini batter, adding more oil to the pan as needed.

6. In a small bowl, mix together the vegan yogurt, lemon juice, dill and salt for the lemon dill sauce.

7. Serve the warm zucchini fritters with the lemon dill sauce on the side. Enjoy!

68. Stuffed Grape Leaves

Ingredient:

- 1 jar (16 oz) grape leaves, rinsed and drained
- 1 cup cooked brown rice
- 1 cup chopped fresh parsley
- 1/2 cup chopped fresh mint
- 1/2 cup chopped onion
- 3 cloves garlic, minced
- 2 tbsp olive oil
- 1 tsp lemon juice
- 1/2 tsp salt
- 1/4 tsp black pepper

For the Lemon Sauce:
- 1/2 cup unsweetened almond milk
- 2 tbsp lemon juice
- 1 tsp cornstarch
- 1/4 tsp salt

Instructions:

1. In a medium bowl, combine the cooked brown rice, parsley, mint, onion, garlic, olive oil, lemon juice, salt and pepper. Mix well.

2. Carefully unroll the grape leaves and place about 1•2 tbsp of the rice mixture near the stem end of each leaf. Fold the sides over the filling and then roll up tightly.

3. Arrange the stuffed grape leaves seam•side down in a large pot. Pour in enough water to just cover the rolls.

4. Bring the water to a boil, then reduce heat and simmer for 30•40 minutes, until the grape leaves are tender.

5. In a small saucepan, whisk together the almond milk, lemon juice, cornstarch and salt for the lemon sauce. Cook over medium heat, stirring constantly, until thickened slightly, about 2•3 minutes.

6. Serve the stuffed grape leaves warm, drizzled with the lemon sauce.

69. Sweet Potato Bites with Guacamole

Ingredient:

For the Sweet Potato Bites:
- 2 medium sweet potatoes, peeled and cut into 1/2•inch thick rounds
- 2 tbsp olive oil
- 1 tsp smoked paprika
- 1/2 tsp garlic powder
- 1/4 tsp salt
- 1/4 tsp black pepper

For the Guacamole:
- 2 ripe avocados, pitted and mashed
- 1/4 cup diced red onion
- 2 tbsp chopped fresh cilantro
- 1 tbsp lime juice
- 1/2 tsp ground cumin
- 1/4 tsp salt

Instructions:

1. Preheat the oven to 400°F. Line a baking sheet with parchment paper.

2. In a large bowl, toss the sweet potato rounds with the olive oil, smoked paprika, garlic powder, salt, and pepper until evenly coated.

3. Arrange the seasoned sweet potato rounds in a single layer on the prepared baking sheet.

4. Bake for 20•25 minutes, flipping halfway, until the sweet potatoes are tender and lightly browned.

5. While the sweet potato bites are baking, make the guacamole. In a medium bowl, mash the avocados with a fork. Stir in the diced red onion, chopped cilantro, lime juice, cumin, and salt. Mix well.

6. Serve the warm sweet potato bites topped with the fresh guacamole.

Enjoy these delicious and nutritious vegan sweet potato bites with creamy guacamole!

70. Mushroom Pâté on Crostini

Ingredient:

For the Mushroom Pâté:
- 1 lb mixed mushrooms (such as cremini, shiitake, and oyster), chopped
- 1 shallot, minced
- 3 cloves garlic, minced
- 2 tbsp olive oil
- 1 tsp dried thyme
- 1/2 tsp dried rosemary
- 1/4 cup raw cashews, soaked in water for at least 2 hours
- 2 tbsp lemon juice
- 1 tsp Dijon mustard
- 1/2 tsp salt
- 1/4 tsp black pepper

For the Crostini:
- 1 baguette, sliced into 1/2•inch thick rounds
- 2 tbsp olive oil

Instructions:

1. In a large skillet, heat the 2 tbsp of olive oil over medium heat. Add the chopped mushrooms, shallot, and garlic. Sauté for 8•10 minutes, until the mushrooms are tender and the liquid has evaporated.

2. Transfer the sautéed mushroom mixture to a food processor. Drain and add the soaked cashews, lemon juice, Dijon mustard, salt, and pepper. Pulse until a smooth pâté•like consistency is achieved, scraping down the sides as needed.

3. Preheat the oven to 400°F. Arrange the baguette slices on a baking sheet and brush both sides lightly with the 2 tbsp of olive oil.

4. Bake the crostini for 5•7 minutes per side, until golden brown and crispy.

5. Spread the mushroom pâté generously onto the crostini. Serve immediately.

Why this is menopause•friendly:
- Mushrooms are a great source of antioxidants, vitamins, and minerals that can help support menopausal health.
- Cashews provide healthy fats and protein to help keep you feeling satisfied.
- Olive oil contains anti•inflammatory monounsaturated fats.

71. Garlic Roasted Brussels Sprouts

Ingredient:

- 1 lb Brussels sprouts, trimmed and halved
- 3 tbsp olive oil
- 4 cloves garlic, minced
- 1 tsp dried thyme
- 1/2 tsp salt
- 1/4 tsp black pepper
- 1 tbsp balsamic vinegar

Instructions:

1. Preheat the oven to 400°F. Line a large baking sheet with parchment paper.

2. In a large bowl, toss the trimmed and halved Brussels sprouts with the olive oil, minced garlic, dried thyme, salt, and black pepper until evenly coated.

3. Spread the seasoned Brussels sprouts in a single layer on the prepared baking sheet.

4. Roast for 20•25 minutes, tossing halfway, until the Brussels sprouts are tender and lightly browned.

5. Remove the roasted Brussels sprouts from the oven and drizzle with the balsamic vinegar. Toss to coat. Serve the garlic roasted Brussels sprouts warm.

Why this is menopause•friendly:

- Brussels sprouts are a cruciferous vegetable that are high in fiber, vitamins, and antioxidants, which can help support menopausal health.

- Garlic has anti•inflammatory properties and may help alleviate some menopausal symptoms.

- Olive oil provides healthy monounsaturated fats that can also help reduce inflammation.

- Balsamic vinegar is a natural diuretic, which can help with water retention.

- The overall dish is low in calories and carbs, while still being flavorful and satisfying.

Enjoy these delicious and nutritious vegan garlic roasted Brussels sprouts!

72. Quinoa Pilaf with Cranberries

Ingredient:

- 1 cup uncooked quinoa, rinsed
- 2 cups vegetable broth
- 1/2 cup dried cranberries
- 1/4 cup chopped fresh parsley
- 2 tbsp olive oil
- 1 shallot, minced
- 2 cloves garlic, minced
- 1 tsp ground cumin
- 1/2 tsp ground coriander
- 1/4 tsp salt
- 1/4 tsp black pepper

Instructions:

1. In a medium saucepan, combine the rinsed quinoa and vegetable broth. Bring to a boil, then reduce heat to low, cover and simmer for 15•20 minutes, until the quinoa is tender and the liquid is absorbed.

2. Fluff the cooked quinoa with a fork and transfer to a large bowl. Stir in the dried cranberries and chopped parsley. Set aside.

3. In a small skillet, heat the olive oil over medium heat. Add the minced shallot and garlic. Cook for 2•3 minutes, until fragrant and softened.

4. Add the cooked shallot and garlic to the quinoa mixture. Sprinkle in the ground cumin, coriander, salt and pepper. Stir to combine.

5. Serve the quinoa pilaf warm or at room temperature. Enjoy!

Variations:
- Add toasted nuts or seeds for extra crunch.
- Swap the cranberries for dried cherries or apricots.
- Stir in some roasted vegetables like butternut squash or Brussels sprouts.
- Top with crumbled feta or goat cheese.

This quinoa pilaf makes a great side dish or vegetarian main course. The combination of fluffy quinoa, tart cranberries, and aromatic spices creates a delicious and nutritious meal.

73. Mashed Cauliflower with Chives

Ingredient:

- 1 large head of cauliflower, cut into florets
- 1/2 cup unsweetened almond milk
- 2 tbsp olive oil
- 2 tbsp chopped fresh chives
- 1 tsp garlic powder
- 1/2 tsp salt
- 1/4 tsp black pepper

Instructions:

1. In a large pot, bring 1•2 inches of water to a boil. Add the cauliflower florets, cover and steam for 10•15 minutes, until very tender.

2. Drain the cauliflower and transfer to a food processor or high•powered blender.

3. Add the almond milk, olive oil, chives, garlic powder, salt and pepper. Blend or process until smooth and creamy, scraping down the sides as needed.

4. Taste and adjust seasoning as desired. Add more almond milk for a thinner consistency if needed.

5. Transfer the mashed cauliflower to a serving bowl. Garnish with extra chopped chives if desired. Serve warm.

Why this is menopause•friendly:
• Cauliflower is a great source of fiber, vitamins and minerals that can help manage menopausal symptoms.

• Almond milk is dairy•free and low in calories, making it a good choice for menopausal women.

• Olive oil provides healthy fats that can help reduce inflammation. Chives are a natural diuretic, which can help relieve water retention. The overall dish is low in calories and carbs, while still being satisfying and flavorful.

Enjoy this nutritious and delicious mashed cauliflower side dish!

74. Roasted Beet and Citrus Salad

Ingredient:

- 3 medium beets, peeled and cut into 1•inch cubes
- 2 tbsp olive oil
- 1/4 tsp salt
- 1/8 tsp black pepper
- 1 orange, peeled and segmented
- 1 grapefruit, peeled and segmented
- 1/4 cup toasted walnuts
- 2 tbsp fresh parsley, chopped
- 2 tbsp balsamic vinegar
- 1 tbsp Dijon mustard
- 1 tbsp maple syrup
- 1 tbsp olive oil
- 1/4 tsp salt
- 1/8 tsp black pepper

Instructions:

1. Preheat the oven to 400°F. Line a baking sheet with parchment paper.

2. In a medium bowl, toss the cubed beets with 2 tbsp of olive oil, 1/4 tsp salt, and 1/8 tsp black pepper until evenly coated.

3. Spread the seasoned beets in a single layer on the prepared baking sheet. Roast for 25•30 minutes, tossing halfway, until the beets are tender and lightly caramelized.

4. Remove the roasted beets from the oven and let cool slightly.

5. In a large bowl, combine the roasted beets, orange segments, grapefruit segments, toasted walnuts, and chopped parsley.

6. In a small bowl, whisk together the balsamic vinegar, Dijon mustard, maple syrup, 1 tbsp olive oil, 1/4 tsp salt, and 1/8 tsp black pepper to make the dressing.

7. Drizzle the dressing over the salad and gently toss to coat.

8. Serve the roasted beet and citrus salad chilled or at room temperature.

Enjoy this refreshing and flavorful vegan roasted beet and citrus salad!

75. Sweet Potato Fries with Avocado Dip

Ingredient:

For the Sweet Potato Fries:
- 2 lbs sweet potatoes, peeled and cut into 1/2•inch thick fries
- 2 tbsp olive oil
- 1 tsp garlic powder
- 1/2 tsp smoked paprika
- 1/2 tsp salt
- 1/4 tsp black pepper

For the Avocado Dip:
- 2 ripe avocados, pitted and mashed
- 1/4 cup unsweetened almond milk
- 2 tbsp fresh lime juice
- 2 tbsp chopped fresh cilantro
- 1 clove garlic, minced
- 1/2 tsp ground cumin
- 1/4 tsp salt

Instructions:

1. Preheat the oven to 400°F. Line a large baking sheet with parchment paper.

2. In a large bowl, toss the sweet potato fries with the olive oil, garlic powder, smoked paprika, salt, and black pepper until evenly coated.

3. Spread the seasoned sweet potato fries in a single layer on the prepared baking sheet.

4. Bake for 20•25 minutes, flipping halfway, until the fries are tender and lightly browned.

5. While the fries are baking, make the avocado dip. In a medium bowl, mash the avocados. Stir in the almond milk, lime juice, cilantro, minced garlic, cumin, and salt. Mix well until smooth and creamy. Serve the warm sweet potato fries with the cool avocado dip on the side. Enjoy!

Why this is menopause•friendly:

• Sweet potatoes are high in fiber, vitamins, and antioxidants that can help manage menopausal symptoms. Avocados are rich in healthy fats, which can help reduce inflammation.

76. Steamed Asparagus with Lemon

Ingredient:

- 1 lb fresh asparagus, tough ends trimmed
- 2 tbsp fresh lemon juice
- 1 tbsp olive oil
- 1/2 tsp salt
- 1/4 tsp black pepper
- Zest of 1 lemon
- 2 tbsp chopped fresh parsley (optional)

Instructions:

1. Fill a large pot with about 1 inch of water and bring to a boil over high heat. Place a steamer basket in the pot.

2. Add the trimmed asparagus spears to the steamer basket. Cover and steam for 5•7 minutes, until the asparagus is tender•crisp.

3. Transfer the steamed asparagus to a serving dish. Drizzle with the lemon juice and olive oil. Sprinkle with the salt, black pepper, and lemon zest.

4. Garnish with the chopped fresh parsley, if using.

5. Serve the steamed asparagus warm or at room temperature.

Tips:
- For thicker asparagus spears, steam for 7•9 minutes.

- You can also roast the asparagus instead of steaming. Toss with the lemon juice, oil, salt and pepper, then roast at 400°F for 10•12 minutes.

- Add a squeeze of fresh lemon juice just before serving for an extra bright flavor.

- Sprinkle with toasted slivered almonds or shaved Parmesan cheese for extra flavor and texture.

This simple steamed asparagus dish highlights the fresh, vibrant flavor of the asparagus, complemented by the bright lemon. It's a quick and easy side dish that pairs well with a variety of main courses.

77. Sautéed Green Beans with Almonds

Ingredient:

- 1 lb fresh green beans, trimmed
- 2 tbsp olive oil
- 3 cloves garlic, minced
- 1/4 cup sliced almonds
- 1 tbsp lemon juice
- 1/2 tsp salt
- 1/4 tsp black pepper
- 2 tbsp chopped fresh parsley

Instructions:

1. In a large skillet, heat the olive oil over medium heat. Add the trimmed green beans and sauté for 5•7 minutes, stirring occasionally, until the beans are tender•crisp.

2. Add the minced garlic to the skillet and cook for 1 minute, until fragrant.

3. Stir in the sliced almonds and continue cooking for 2•3 minutes, until the almonds are lightly toasted.

4. Remove the skillet from heat and stir in the lemon juice, salt, and black pepper.

5. Transfer the sautéed green beans and almonds to a serving dish. Sprinkle with the chopped fresh parsley. Serve the green bean almondine warm or at room temperature.

Why this is menopause•friendly:

• Green beans are a great source of fiber, vitamins, and minerals that can help manage menopausal symptoms.

• Almonds provide healthy fats, protein, and antioxidants that can help reduce inflammation.

• Lemon juice is a natural diuretic that can help with water retention.

• Parsley is a natural herb that may help alleviate some menopausal symptoms.

• Olive oil contains anti•inflammatory monounsaturated fats. The overall dish is low in calories and carbs, making it a nutritious option for menopausal women.

78. Wild Rice Salad with Pecans

Ingredient:

- 1 cup uncooked wild rice
- 3 cups vegetable broth
- 1/2 cup chopped pecans
- 1/2 cup dried cranberries
- 1/2 cup diced celery
- 1/4 cup diced red onion
- 2 tbsp chopped fresh parsley
- 2 tbsp olive oil
- 2 tbsp apple cider vinegar
- 1 tbsp Dijon mustard
- 1 tsp maple syrup
- 1/2 tsp salt
- 1/4 tsp black pepper

Instructions:

1. In a medium saucepan, combine the wild rice and vegetable broth. Bring to a boil, then reduce heat to low, cover and simmer for 45•50 minutes, until the rice is tender and the liquid is absorbed. Fluff with a fork and let cool.

2. In a large bowl, combine the cooked wild rice, chopped pecans, dried cranberries, diced celery, diced red onion, and chopped parsley.

3. In a small bowl, whisk together the olive oil, apple cider vinegar, Dijon mustard, maple syrup, salt, and black pepper to make the dressing.

4. Pour the dressing over the wild rice salad and toss gently to coat.

5. Serve the wild rice salad chilled or at room temperature. Enjoy!

Variations:
- Add diced apples or pears for extra sweetness.
- Swap the pecans for walnuts or almonds.
- Use dried cherries or raisins instead of cranberries.
- Stir in some crumbled feta or goat cheese.

This wild rice salad makes a great side dish or light main course. The nutty wild rice, crunchy pecans, and tangy•sweet dressing create a delicious and nutritious meal.

79. Vegan Coleslaw with Apple Cider Vinegar

Ingredient:

- 1 head green cabbage, shredded (about 6 cups)
- 1 carrot, grated (about 1 cup)
- 1/2 red onion, thinly sliced
- 1/2 cup vegan mayonnaise (or plain unsweetened vegan yogurt)
- 2 tbsp apple cider vinegar
- 1 tbsp Dijon mustard
- 1 tbsp maple syrup
- 1/2 tsp salt
- 1/4 tsp black pepper

Instructions:

1. In a large bowl, combine the shredded green cabbage, grated carrot, and sliced red onion. Toss to mix.

2. In a small bowl, whisk together the vegan mayonnaise, apple cider vinegar, Dijon mustard, maple syrup, salt, and black pepper to make the dressing.

3. Pour the dressing over the cabbage mixture and toss gently to coat everything evenly.

4. Cover and refrigerate the coleslaw for at least 30 minutes, or up to 3 days, to allow the flavors to meld.

5. Serve the vegan coleslaw chilled or at room temperature.

Variations:
- Add shredded kale or Brussels sprouts for extra crunch and nutrition.

- Stir in chopped apples, pineapple, or raisins for a sweet twist.

- Top with toasted sunflower seeds or sliced almonds.

- Use a combination of green and red cabbage for more color.

The apple cider vinegar in the dressing gives this vegan coleslaw a nice tangy flavor that balances the sweetness of the maple syrup. It's a refreshing and healthy side dish that pairs well with burgers, sandwiches, or barbecue.

80. Roasted Butternut Squash with Sage

Ingredient:

- 1 medium butternut squash, peeled, seeded and cut into 1•inch cubes (about 4 cups)
- 2 tbsp olive oil
- 1 tsp dried sage
- 1/2 tsp salt
- 1/4 tsp black pepper
- 2 tbsp chopped fresh sage leaves

Instructions:

1. Preheat the oven to 400°F. Line a large baking sheet with parchment paper.

2. In a large bowl, toss the cubed butternut squash with the olive oil, dried sage, salt, and black pepper until the squash is evenly coated.

3. Spread the seasoned squash in a single layer on the prepared baking sheet.

4. Roast for 25•30 minutes, flipping the squash halfway, until it is tender and lightly browned.

5. Remove the roasted butternut squash from the oven and transfer to a serving dish.

6. Sprinkle the chopped fresh sage leaves over the top of the roasted squash.

7. Serve the roasted butternut squash with sage warm or at room temperature.

Variations:
- Add a sprinkle of grated Parmesan cheese or crumbled feta for extra flavor.

- Toss the roasted squash with toasted pumpkin seeds or chopped walnuts.

- Drizzle with a balsamic glaze or maple syrup for a sweet•savory contrast.

- Use other fresh herbs like thyme or rosemary in place of the sage.

The combination of sweet, caramelized butternut squash and fragrant, earthy sage makes this a delicious and easy side dish. Enjoy the warm, comforting flavors of this roasted squash recipe.

81. Tomato Basil Soup

Ingredient:

- 2 tbsp olive oil
- 1 onion, diced
- 3 cloves garlic, minced
- 1 tsp dried oregano
- 1/2 tsp dried thyme
- 1/4 tsp red pepper flakes (optional)
- 1 (28oz) can diced tomatoes
- 2 cups low•sodium vegetable broth
- 1 (15oz) can white beans, drained and rinsed
- 1/4 cup fresh basil leaves, chopped
- 1 tbsp balsamic vinegar
- 1 tsp salt
- 1/4 tsp black pepper
- 1/2 cup unsweetened almond milk

Instructions:

1. In a large pot, heat the olive oil over medium heat. Add the diced onion and sauté for 5•7 minutes until translucent.

2. Add the minced garlic, dried oregano, thyme, and red pepper flakes (if using). Cook for 1 minute, stirring constantly, until fragrant.

3. Pour in the canned diced tomatoes and vegetable broth. Bring the mixture to a simmer.

4. Stir in the drained and rinsed white beans, chopped fresh basil, balsamic vinegar, salt, and black pepper.

5. Reduce heat to medium•low and let the soup simmer for 15•20 minutes, allowing the flavors to meld.

6. Remove the pot from heat and use an immersion blender to partially purée the soup, leaving some texture. Alternatively, you can carefully transfer batches to a blender.

7. Stir in the unsweetened almond milk and adjust seasoning as needed.

8. Serve the tomato basil soup warm, garnished with extra fresh basil if desired.

Enjoy this delicious and nutritious vegan tomato basil soup!

82. Butternut Squash Soup

Ingredient:

- 1 medium butternut squash, peeled, seeded and cubed (about 4 cups)
- 1 tbsp olive oil
- 1 onion, diced
- 3 cloves garlic, minced
- 4 cups low•sodium vegetable broth
- 1 cup unsweetened almond milk
- 1 tsp ground cumin
- 1/2 tsp ground cinnamon
- 1/2 tsp salt
- 1/4 tsp black pepper
- Chopped fresh parsley for garnish (optional)

Instructions:

1. In a large pot or Dutch oven, heat the olive oil over medium heat. Add the diced onion and sauté for 5•7 minutes until translucent.

2. Add the minced garlic and cubed butternut squash. Cook for 2•3 minutes, stirring frequently, until fragrant.

3. Pour in the vegetable broth and almond milk. Bring the mixture to a boil.

4. Reduce heat to medium•low and let the soup simmer for 20•25 minutes, until the squash is very tender.

5. Using an immersion blender, carefully purée the soup until smooth and creamy. Alternatively, you can carefully transfer the soup in batches to a blender.

6. Stir in the ground cumin, cinnamon, salt, and black pepper. Taste and adjust seasoning as needed.

7. Serve the butternut squash soup warm, garnished with chopped fresh parsley if desired.

Variations:
- For a creamier soup, stir in 1/4 cup heavy cream or coconut milk at the end.
- Top with roasted pumpkin seeds, croutons, or a drizzle of pesto.
- Add a pinch of nutmeg or cayenne pepper for extra warmth.
- Swap the almond milk for regular milk or vegetable broth.

83. Carrot Ginger Soup

Ingredient:

- 2 tbsp olive oil
- 1 onion, diced
- 3 cloves garlic, minced
- 1 tbsp grated fresh ginger
- 1 lb carrots, peeled and chopped
- 4 cups low•sodium vegetable broth
- 1 (13.5 oz) can full•fat coconut milk
- 1 tsp ground turmeric
- 1/2 tsp ground cumin
- 1/2 tsp salt
- 1/4 tsp black pepper
- 2 tbsp fresh lemon juice
- Chopped fresh cilantro for garnish (optional)

Instructions:

1. In a large pot, heat the olive oil over medium heat. Add the diced onion and sauté for 5•7 minutes until translucent.

2. Add the minced garlic and grated ginger. Cook for 1 minute, stirring constantly, until fragrant.

3. Stir in the chopped carrots, vegetable broth, coconut milk, turmeric, cumin, salt, and black pepper. Bring the soup to a boil.

4. Reduce heat to medium•low and let the soup simmer for 20•25 minutes, until the carrots are very tender.

5. Using an immersion blender, carefully purée the soup until smooth and creamy. Alternatively, you can carefully transfer the soup in batches to a blender.

6. Stir in the fresh lemon juice and adjust seasoning as needed.

7. Serve the carrot ginger soup warm, garnished with chopped fresh cilantro if desired.

Enjoy this comforting and nourishing vegan carrot ginger soup!

84. Minestrone with Beans

Ingredient:

- 2 tbsp olive oil
- 1 onion, diced
- 3 cloves garlic, minced
- 2 carrots, peeled and diced
- 2 celery stalks, diced
- 1 zucchini, diced
- 1 (15oz) can diced tomatoes
- 4 cups low•sodium vegetable broth
- 1 (15oz) can kidney beans, drained and rinsed
- 1 (15oz) can white beans, drained and rinsed
- 2 cups chopped kale or spinach
- 1 tsp dried oregano
- 1 tsp dried basil
- 1/2 tsp salt
- 1/4 tsp black pepper
- 2 tbsp chopped fresh parsley
- 1 tbsp lemon juice

Instructions:

1. In a large pot, heat the olive oil over medium heat. Add the diced onion and sauté for 5 minutes until translucent.

2. Stir in the minced garlic, diced carrots, celery, and zucchini. Cook for 3•4 minutes, until the vegetables start to soften.

3. Pour in the canned diced tomatoes and vegetable broth. Bring the soup to a boil.

4. Reduce heat to medium•low and stir in the drained and rinsed kidney and white beans, chopped kale/spinach, dried oregano, dried basil, salt, and black pepper.

5. Simmer the minestrone soup for 15•20 minutes, until the vegetables are tender.

6. Remove from heat and stir in the chopped fresh parsley and lemon juice.

7. Serve the minestrone soup hot, garnished with extra parsley if desired.

Enjoy this comforting and nourishing vegan minestrone soup!

85. Miso Soup with Tofu

Ingredient:

- 4 cups low•sodium vegetable broth
- 2 tbsp white or yellow miso paste
- 1 (12oz) block firm or extra•firm tofu, cubed
- 1 cup sliced shiitake mushrooms
- 1 cup chopped bok choy or spinach
- 2 green onions, sliced
- 1 tsp grated fresh ginger
- 1 tsp sesame oil
- 1/4 tsp salt

Instructions:

1. In a medium saucepan, bring the vegetable broth to a gentle simmer over medium heat.

2. In a small bowl, whisk together the miso paste with a few tablespoons of the hot broth until smooth. Pour the miso mixture back into the saucepan, stirring to combine.

3. Add the cubed tofu, sliced shiitake mushrooms, chopped bok choy or spinach, sliced green onions, and grated ginger to the broth.

4. Simmer the miso soup for 5•7 minutes, until the vegetables are tender.

5. Remove the pot from heat and stir in the sesame oil and salt. Ladle the miso soup into bowls and serve hot.

Why this is menopause•friendly:

• Tofu is a great source of plant•based protein that can help maintain muscle mass during menopause.

• Miso is a fermented soy product that contains probiotics to support gut health. Shiitake mushrooms are rich in antioxidants that may help reduce inflammation.

• Bok choy and spinach are nutrient•dense greens that can help manage menopausal symptoms. Ginger has anti•inflammatory properties and may help alleviate hot flashes.

• Sesame oil provides healthy fats that can help keep you feeling full and satisfied. The overall soup is low in calories and carbs, making it a nutritious option for menopausal women.

86. Sweet Potato and Lentil Soup

Ingredient:

- 1 tbsp olive oil
- 1 onion, diced
- 3 cloves garlic, minced
- 1 tsp ground cumin
- 1 tsp ground coriander
- 1/2 tsp smoked paprika
- 1/4 tsp cayenne pepper (optional)
- 4 cups low•sodium vegetable broth
- 1 cup red lentils, rinsed
- 2 medium sweet potatoes, peeled and cubed
- 1 (14oz) can diced tomatoes
- 1 tsp salt
- 1/4 tsp black pepper
- 2 cups baby spinach, chopped
- 2 tbsp fresh lemon juice

Instructions:

1. In a large pot, heat the olive oil over medium heat. Add the diced onion and sauté for 5 minutes until translucent.

2. Add the minced garlic, cumin, coriander, smoked paprika, and cayenne (if using). Cook for 1 minute, stirring constantly, until fragrant.

3. Pour in the vegetable broth and add the rinsed lentils and cubed sweet potatoes. Bring to a boil.

4. Reduce heat to medium•low and simmer for 20•25 minutes, until the lentils and sweet potatoes are tender.

5. Stir in the diced tomatoes, salt, and black pepper. Cook for 5 more minutes.

6. Remove from heat and stir in the chopped spinach and lemon juice.

7. Serve the sweet potato and lentil soup hot, garnished with extra lemon wedges if desired.

Enjoy this comforting and nourishing vegan sweet potato and lentil soup!

87. Creamy Broccoli Soup

Ingredient:

- 2 tbsp olive oil
- 1 onion, diced
- 3 cloves garlic, minced
- 1 lb broccoli florets, chopped
- 4 cups low•sodium vegetable broth
- 1 cup unsweetened almond milk
- 2 tbsp tahini
- 1 tsp ground turmeric
- 1 tsp ground cumin
- 1/2 tsp ground ginger
- Salt and pepper to taste
- Chopped parsley for garnish

Instructions:

1. In a large pot, heat the olive oil over medium heat. Add the onion and sauté for 5 minutes until translucent.

2. Add the garlic and sauté for 1 minute until fragrant.

3. Add the chopped broccoli florets and vegetable broth. Bring to a boil, then reduce heat and simmer for 10•15 minutes, until the broccoli is very tender.

4. Remove from heat and use an immersion blender to puree the soup until smooth and creamy.

5. Stir in the almond milk, tahini, turmeric, cumin, and ginger. Season with salt and pepper to taste.

6. Return the soup to low heat and cook for 5 more minutes, stirring occasionally, until heated through.

7. Ladle the soup into bowls and garnish with chopped parsley.

This creamy broccoli soup is packed with nutrients that can help support women during menopause, including fiber, antioxidants, and anti•inflammatory compounds. The tahini and almond milk provide a creamy texture without dairy. Enjoy this comforting and nourishing soup!

88. Vegan Pho with Rice Noodles

Ingredient:

- 8 oz rice noodles
- 6 cups vegetable broth
- 2 tablespoons soy sauce or tamari
- 1 tablespoon rice vinegar
- 1 teaspoon sesame oil
- 1 teaspoon ground coriander
- 1 teaspoon ground cumin
- 1/2 teaspoon ground ginger
- 1/4 teaspoon ground turmeric
- 2 cups sliced mushrooms
- 1 cup thinly sliced carrots
- 1 cup thinly sliced bok choy or other leafy green
- 1/2 cup thinly sliced red onion
- 2 cloves garlic, minced
- 1 jalapeño, thinly sliced (optional)
- Chopped cilantro, lime wedges, and sriracha for serving

Instructions:

1. Prepare the rice noodles according to package instructions. Drain and set aside.

2. In a large pot, combine the vegetable broth, soy sauce, rice vinegar, sesame oil, coriander, cumin, ginger, and turmeric. Bring to a simmer over medium heat.

3. Add the mushrooms, carrots, bok choy, red onion, and garlic. Simmer for 5•7 minutes, until the vegetables are tender.

4. Add the cooked rice noodles to the pot and heat through, about 2•3 minutes.

5. Serve the pho hot, garnished with chopped cilantro, lime wedges, and a drizzle of sriracha (if desired).

This vegan pho is packed with nutrient•dense vegetables and soothing spices that can help alleviate some of the common symptoms associated with menopause, such as hot flashes, mood swings, and joint pain. The rice noodles provide a satisfying base, while the broth and toppings offer a flavorful and comforting meal.

89. Split Pea Soup with Carrots

Ingredient:

- 1 tbsp olive oil
- 1 onion, diced
- 3 cloves garlic, minced
- 1 lb split peas, rinsed
- 6 cups low•sodium vegetable broth
- 3 carrots, peeled and diced
- 1 tsp ground cumin
- 1 tsp ground turmeric
- 1/2 tsp ground ginger
- Salt and pepper to taste
- Chopped parsley for garnish

Instructions:

1. In a large pot, heat the olive oil over medium heat. Add the diced onion and sauté for 5•7 minutes until translucent.

2. Add the minced garlic and sauté for 1 minute until fragrant.

3. Stir in the rinsed split peas and vegetable broth. Bring the mixture to a boil.

4. Reduce heat to low, cover, and let the soup simmer for 30•40 minutes, stirring occasionally, until the split peas are very soft.

5. Add the diced carrots, cumin, turmeric, and ginger. Season with salt and pepper to taste.

6. Continue simmering the soup for 15•20 minutes, until the carrots are tender.

7. Use an immersion blender to partially puree the soup, leaving some texture.

8. Ladle the split pea soup into bowls and garnish with chopped parsley.

This vegan split pea soup is packed with fiber, protein, and nutrients that can help support women during menopause. The carrots provide beta•carotene and the spices offer anti•inflammatory benefits. Enjoy this comforting and nourishing soup!

90. Zucchini and Leek Soup

Ingredient:

- 2 tbsp olive oil
- 2 leeks, white and light green parts only, thinly sliced
- 3 zucchini, chopped
- 4 cups low•sodium vegetable broth
- 1 cup unsweetened almond milk
- 2 tbsp tahini
- 1 tsp ground turmeric
- 1 tsp ground cumin
- 1/2 tsp ground ginger
- Salt and pepper to taste
- Chopped parsley for garnish

Instructions:

1. In a large pot, heat the olive oil over medium heat. Add the sliced leeks and sauté for 5•7 minutes, until softened.

2. Add the chopped zucchini and continue cooking for 3•4 minutes.

3. Pour in the vegetable broth and bring the mixture to a boil. Reduce heat and let simmer for 10•15 minutes, until the zucchini is very tender.

4. Remove the pot from heat and use an immersion blender to puree the soup until smooth and creamy.

5. Stir in the almond milk, tahini, turmeric, cumin, and ginger. Season with salt and pepper to taste.

6. Return the soup to low heat and cook for 5 more minutes, stirring occasionally, until heated through.

7. Ladle the soup into bowls and garnish with chopped parsley.

This vegan zucchini and leek soup is a nourishing and comforting option for women during menopause. The zucchini provides fiber, vitamins, and antioxidants, while the leeks, tahini, and spices offer anti•inflammatory benefits. The almond milk makes it creamy without dairy. Enjoy this soothing and flavorful soup!

91. Vegan Lasagna with Cashew Ricotta

Ingredient:

For the Cashew Ricotta:
- 1 cup raw cashews, soaked in water
  for at least 4 hours or overnight
- 1/4 cup unsweetened almond milk
- 2 tbsp lemon juice
- 1 tsp apple cider vinegar
- 1/2 tsp salt

For the Lasagna:
- 9 lasagna noodles
- 1 tbsp olive oil
- 1 onion, diced
- 3 cloves garlic, minced
- 1 (28oz) can crushed tomatoes
- 2 tsp dried oregano
- 1 tsp dried basil
- 1/2 tsp salt
- 1/4 tsp black pepper
- 1 (15oz) can diced tomatoes
- 1 (15oz) can kidney beans, drained and rinsed
- 1 (10oz) package frozen spinach, thawed and drained

Instructions:

1. Make the cashew ricotta: Drain and rinse the soaked cashews. Add them to a food processor along with the almond milk, lemon juice, apple cider vinegar, and salt. Blend until smooth and creamy. Set aside.

2. Preheat the oven to 375°F. Cook the lasagna noodles according to package instructions. Drain and set aside.

3. In a large skillet, heat the olive oil over medium heat. Add the diced onion and sauté for 5 minutes until translucent. Stir in the minced garlic and cook for 1 minute.

4. Add the crushed tomatoes, dried oregano, dried basil, salt, and black pepper. Simmer for 10 minutes.

5. Stir in the diced tomatoes, drained and rinsed kidney beans, and thawed spinach. Cook for 5 more minutes. Spread 1 cup of the tomato•bean•spinach mixture in the bottom of a 9x13 inch baking dish. Top with 3 lasagna noodles.

6. Spread half of the cashew ricotta over the noodles, then top with another layer of 3 noodles. Spread the remaining tomato•bean•spinach mixture over the noodles, then top with the final 3 noodles.

7. Spread the remaining cashew ricotta over the top.. Cover the dish with foil and bake for 30 minutes. Remove the foil and bake for an additional 15 minutes. Let the lasagna cool for 10•15 minutes before slicing and serving.

92. Moroccan Chickpea Stew

Ingredient:

- 2 tbsp olive oil
- 1 onion, diced
- 3 cloves garlic, minced
- 1 tbsp ground cumin
- 1 tsp ground coriander
- 1 tsp ground turmeric
- 1/2 tsp ground cinnamon
- 1/4 tsp cayenne pepper (optional)
- 1 (15oz) can diced tomatoes
- 1 (15oz) can chickpeas, drained and rinsed
- 3 cups low•sodium vegetable broth
- 1 medium sweet potato, peeled and cubed
- 1 cup chopped cauliflower florets
- 1 cup chopped kale or spinach
- Salt and pepper to taste
- Chopped cilantro for garnish

Instructions:

1. In a large pot, heat the olive oil over medium heat. Add the diced onion and sauté for 5•7 minutes until translucent.

2. Add the minced garlic and spices (cumin, coriander, turmeric, cinnamon, cayenne if using). Sauté for 1•2 minutes until fragrant.

3. Stir in the diced tomatoes, drained chickpeas, and vegetable broth. Bring the mixture to a boil.

4. Add the cubed sweet potato and cauliflower florets. Reduce heat to low, cover, and simmer for 15•20 minutes, until the vegetables are tender.

5. Stir in the chopped kale or spinach and cook for 2•3 minutes until wilted.

6. Season the stew with salt and pepper to taste. Ladle the Moroccan chickpea stew into bowls and garnish with chopped cilantro.

This vegan Moroccan chickpea stew is packed with fiber, protein, and anti•inflammatory spices that can help support women during menopause. The sweet potato, cauliflower, and leafy greens provide a nutrient•dense base. Enjoy this flavorful and comforting stew!

93. Ratatouille with Polenta

Ingredient:

Ratatouille:
- 2 tbsp olive oil
- 1 eggplant, diced
- 1 zucchini, diced
- 1 yellow squash, diced
- 1 red bell pepper, diced
- 1 onion, diced
- 3 cloves garlic, minced
- 1 (14oz) can diced tomatoes
- 2 tsp dried oregano
- 1 tsp dried thyme
- Salt and pepper to taste
- Chopped basil for garnish

Polenta:
- 4 cups low•sodium vegetable broth
- 1 cup polenta or cornmeal
- 2 tbsp tahini
- 1 tsp ground turmeric
- Salt and pepper to taste

Instructions:

For the Ratatouille:
1. In a large skillet, heat the olive oil over medium heat. Add the diced eggplant, zucchini, yellow squash, bell pepper, and onion. Sauté for 8•10 minutes until vegetables are tender.
2. Add the minced garlic and sauté for 1 minute until fragrant.
3. Stir in the diced tomatoes, oregano, and thyme. Season with salt and pepper.
4. Reduce heat to low and let the ratatouille simmer for 15•20 minutes, stirring occasionally, until the flavors have melded.

For the Polenta:
1. In a medium saucepan, bring the vegetable broth to a boil over high heat.
2. Slowly whisk in the polenta. Reduce heat to low and let the polenta simmer, stirring frequently, for 15•20 minutes until thickened.
3. Remove from heat and stir in the tahini and turmeric. Season with salt and pepper.

To Serve:
1. Spoon the warm polenta into bowls.
2. Top with the ratatouille and garnish with chopped basil.

This vegan ratatouille with polenta is a nourishing and comforting meal tailored for menopause. The vegetables provide fiber, antioxidants, and anti•inflammatory benefits, while the polenta offers complex carbs and the tahini provides healthy fats.

94. Vegan Paella with Artichokes

Ingredient:

- 1 cup short•grain brown rice
- 3 cups low•sodium vegetable broth
- 2 tbsp olive oil
- 1 onion, diced
- 3 cloves garlic, minced
- 1 tsp smoked paprika
- 1/2 tsp saffron threads (optional)
- 1 cup frozen artichoke hearts, thawed and halved
- 1 cup diced tomatoes
- 1 cup frozen peas
- 1 cup cooked chickpeas, rinsed and drained
- 1/4 cup chopped fresh parsley
- 1 tbsp lemon juice
- 1/2 tsp salt
- 1/4 tsp black pepper

Instructions:

1. In a medium saucepan, combine the brown rice and vegetable broth. Bring to a boil, then reduce heat to low, cover and simmer for 40•45 minutes, until the rice is tender. Fluff with a fork.

2. In a large skillet or paella pan, heat the olive oil over medium heat. Add the diced onion and sauté for 5 minutes until translucent.

3. Stir in the minced garlic, smoked paprika, and saffron (if using). Cook for 1 minute, until fragrant.

4. Add the thawed and halved artichoke hearts, diced tomatoes, frozen peas, and cooked chickpeas. Sauté for 5•7 minutes.

5. Stir in the cooked brown rice, chopped parsley, lemon juice, salt, and black pepper. Toss everything together until well combined.

6. Reduce heat to low and let the paella simmer for 5•10 minutes, allowing the flavors to meld.

7. Serve the vegan paella warm, garnished with extra parsley if desired.

95. Cauliflower Steak with Chimichurri

Ingredient:

- 1 large head of cauliflower, cut into 1•inch thick "steaks"
- 2 tbsp olive oil
- Salt and pepper to taste

For the Chimichurri Sauce:
- 1 cup packed fresh parsley leaves
- 3 garlic cloves
- 2 tbsp red wine vinegar
- 1 tbsp fresh oregano leaves
- 1/4 cup olive oil
- 1 tsp red pepper flakes
- Salt and pepper to taste

Instructions:

1. Make the chimichurri sauce. In a food processor, combine the parsley, garlic, red wine vinegar, oregano, olive oil, and red pepper flakes. Pulse until well combined but still a bit chunky. Season with salt and pepper to taste. Set aside.

2. Preheat oven to 400°F. Line a baking sheet with parchment paper.

3. Brush the cauliflower "steaks" on both sides with olive oil and season generously with salt and pepper.

4. Arrange the cauliflower steaks in a single layer on the prepared baking sheet.

5. Roast for 20•25 minutes, flipping halfway, until the cauliflower is tender and lightly browned.

6. Serve the roasted cauliflower steaks immediately, drizzled with the chimichurri sauce. Enjoy!

96. Tempeh Stir•fry with Broccoli

Ingredient:

- 8 oz tempeh, cut into 1•inch cubes
- 2 tbsp sesame oil
- 1 head of broccoli, cut into florets
- 1 red bell pepper, sliced
- 3 cloves garlic, minced
- 1 inch fresh ginger, grated
- 2 tbsp low•sodium soy sauce or tamari
- 1 tbsp rice vinegar
- 1 tsp sesame seeds
- Salt and pepper to taste

For the Sauce:
- 2 tbsp low•sodium soy sauce or tamari
- 1 tbsp rice vinegar
- 1 tsp maple syrup
- 1 tsp arrowroot powder

Instructions:

1. In a small bowl, whisk together the sauce ingredients and set aside.

2. Heat the sesame oil in a large skillet or wok over medium•high heat. Add the tempeh cubes and sauté for 5•7 minutes, until lightly browned on all sides. Remove tempeh from the pan and set aside.

3. Add the broccoli florets and bell pepper slices to the pan. Sauté for 3•4 minutes, until starting to soften.

4. Add the garlic and ginger to the pan and sauté for 1 minute, until fragrant.

5. Pour the sauce mixture into the pan and let it simmer for 2•3 minutes, until thickened slightly.

6. Add the sautéed tempeh back to the pan and toss everything together to coat in the sauce.

7. Remove from heat and sprinkle with sesame seeds. Season with salt and pepper to taste. Serve immediately over steamed brown rice or quinoa. Enjoy!

97. Vegan Pad Thai with Peanut Sauce

Ingredient:

Pad Thai:

- 8 oz rice noodles
- 2 tbsp sesame oil
- 1 block extra•firm tofu, cubed
- 2 cups shredded cabbage
- 1 cup bean sprouts
- 1/2 cup chopped scallions
- 1/4 cup chopped cilantro

Peanut Sauce:

- 1/2 cup creamy peanut butter
- 2 tbsp low•sodium soy sauce or tamari
- 2 tbsp rice vinegar
- 1 tbsp maple syrup
- 1 tsp sesame oil
- 1 tsp ground ginger
- 1/4 tsp cayenne pepper (optional)
- 1/4 cup warm water

Instructions:

1. Prepare the rice noodles according to package instructions. Drain and set aside.

2. In a large skillet or wok, heat the sesame oil over medium•high heat. Add the cubed tofu and sauté for 5•7 minutes until lightly browned on all sides.

3. Add the shredded cabbage, bean sprouts, and scallions to the skillet. Sauté for 2•3 minutes until the vegetables are slightly softened.

4. Add the cooked rice noodles and toss everything together until well combined and heated through.

For the Peanut Sauce:
1. In a medium bowl, whisk together the peanut butter, soy sauce, rice vinegar, maple syrup, sesame oil, ginger, and cayenne (if using).
2. Gradually whisk in the warm water until the sauce is smooth and creamy.

To Serve:
1. Divide the Pad Thai noodle mixture evenly among serving bowls.
2. Drizzle the peanut sauce over the top and garnish with chopped cilantro.

This vegan Pad Thai is a flavorful and nutrient•dense meal that can help support women during menopause. The peanut sauce provides healthy fats, while the tofu, vegetables, and rice noodles offer fiber, protein, and complex carbs. Enjoy this delicious and satisfying dish!

98. Stuffed Acorn Squash

Ingredient:

- 2 acorn squash, halved and seeded
- 2 tbsp olive oil
- 1 cup cooked quinoa
- 1 cup cooked brown rice
- 1 cup diced mushrooms
- 1 cup diced bell pepper
- 1 cup diced onion
- 3 cloves garlic, minced
- 1 tsp dried thyme
- 1 tsp dried sage
- 1/4 cup chopped walnuts
- 2 tbsp pumpkin seeds
- Salt and pepper to taste

For the Sauce:
- 1/4 cup tahini
- 2 tbsp lemon juice
- 2 tbsp water
- 1 tsp maple syrup
- 1/4 tsp ground cumin
- Salt and pepper to taste

Instructions:

1. Preheat oven to 400°F. Place the acorn squash halves cut•side up on a baking sheet. Brush with 1 tbsp of the olive oil and season with salt and pepper. Roast for 30•40 minutes, until tender.

2. In a large skillet, heat the remaining 1 tbsp of olive oil over medium heat. Add the mushrooms, bell pepper, and onion. Sauté for 5•7 minutes, until softened.

3. Add the garlic, thyme, and sage. Sauté for 1 minute more, until fragrant.

4. Remove the skillet from heat and stir in the cooked quinoa and brown rice. Season with salt and pepper.

5. Scoop the quinoa•rice mixture into the roasted acorn squash halves, packing it in tightly.

6. Sprinkle the walnuts and pumpkin seeds over the top of the stuffed squash.

7. In a small bowl, whisk together all the sauce ingredients until smooth. Drizzle the sauce over the stuffed squash.

8. Return the stuffed squash to the oven and bake for an additional 10•15 minutes, until heated through.

9. Serve warm. Enjoy!

99. Seitan Tacos with Cabbage Slaw

Ingredient:

For the Seitan:
- 1 cup vital wheat gluten
- 1/4 cup chickpea flour
- 1 tsp garlic powder
- 1 tsp onion powder
- 1 tsp cumin
- 1/2 tsp smoked paprika
- 1/2 tsp salt
- 1 cup vegetable broth

For Serving:
- 8•10 small corn tortillas, warmed
- Diced avocado
- Lime wedges

For the Cabbage Slaw:
- 2 cups shredded green cabbage
- 1 cup shredded red cabbage
- 1/2 cup shredded carrots
- 1/4 cup chopped cilantro
- 2 tbsp apple cider vinegar
- 1 tbsp olive oil
- 1 tsp Dijon mustard
- 1/2 tsp salt
- 1/4 tsp black pepper

Instructions:

1. Make the seitan: In a large bowl, whisk together the vital wheat gluten, chickpea flour, garlic powder, onion powder, cumin, smoked paprika, and salt. Gradually add the vegetable broth, mixing until a dough forms. Knead the dough for 2•3 minutes.

2. Tear off pieces of the seitan dough and shape into small "meat" patties or crumbles.

3. In a large skillet over medium heat, cook the seitan pieces for 5•7 minutes per side, until browned and slightly crispy.

4. Make the cabbage slaw: In a large bowl, combine the shredded green and red cabbage, shredded carrots, and chopped cilantro.

5. In a small bowl, whisk together the apple cider vinegar, olive oil, Dijon mustard, salt, and black pepper. Pour the dressing over the cabbage mixture and toss to coat.

6. To serve, place the warm corn tortillas on plates and top with the cooked seitan, cabbage slaw, diced avocado, and a squeeze of lime juice.

Enjoy these flavorful and satisfying seitan tacos with a fresh and crunchy cabbage slaw!

100. Vegan Bolognese with Lentils

Ingredient:

- 1 cup dry brown or green lentils, rinsed
- 3 cups vegetable broth
- 2 tbsp olive oil
- 1 onion, diced
- 3 cloves garlic, minced
- 1 carrot, peeled and diced
- 1 celery stalk, diced
- 1 (28 oz) can crushed tomatoes
- 2 tbsp tomato paste
- 1 tsp dried oregano
- 1 tsp dried basil
- 1/4 tsp red pepper flakes (optional)
- Salt and pepper to taste
- Cooked pasta, for serving

Instructions:

1. In a medium saucepan, combine the lentils and vegetable broth. Bring to a boil, then reduce heat and simmer for 15•20 minutes, until lentils are tender. Drain any excess liquid and set aside.

2. In a large skillet, heat the olive oil over medium heat. Add the onion, garlic, carrot, and celery. Sauté for 5•7 minutes, until vegetables are softened.

3. Stir in the cooked lentils, crushed tomatoes, tomato paste, oregano, basil, and red pepper flakes (if using). Season with salt and pepper.

4. Reduce heat to low and let the bolognese simmer for 15•20 minutes, stirring occasionally, to allow the flavors to meld.

5. Serve the vegan bolognese sauce over cooked pasta of your choice. Top with additional fresh basil or parsley if desired.

This hearty, plant•based bolognese is a delicious and nutritious alternative to the traditional meat•based version. The lentils provide a great source of protein, fiber, and other essential nutrients. Enjoy!

101. Spinach Salad with Strawberries and Pecans

Ingredient:

- 5 oz baby spinach
- 1 cup sliced fresh strawberries
- 1/2 cup toasted pecans, chopped
- 2 tbsp balsamic vinegar
- 1 tbsp olive oil
- 1 tsp Dijon mustard
- 1 tsp maple syrup
- Salt and pepper to taste

Instructions:

1. In a large salad bowl, combine the baby spinach, sliced strawberries, and chopped pecans.

2. In a small bowl, whisk together the balsamic vinegar, olive oil, Dijon mustard, and maple syrup. Season with salt and pepper.

3. Drizzle the dressing over the salad and toss gently to coat.

4. Serve immediately. Enjoy!

The key menopause•friendly ingredients in this recipe are:

• Spinach • a nutrient•dense leafy green that is high in calcium, folate, and magnesium

• Strawberries • a fruit that is rich in antioxidants and phytoestrogens

• Pecans • a good source of healthy fats, including omega•3 fatty acids

• Maple syrup • a natural sweetener that is lower in glycemic index than refined sugar

This salad is a great source of fiber, vitamins, and minerals that can help support women during menopause. The combination of the nutrient•rich spinach, sweet strawberries, and crunchy pecans makes for a delicious and satisfying meal.

102. Arugula Salad with Beets and Walnuts

Ingredient:

- 5 oz baby arugula
- 2 medium beets, roasted and diced
- 1/2 cup toasted walnuts, chopped
- 2 tbsp crumbled feta cheese (optional)
- 2 tbsp olive oil
- 1 tbsp balsamic vinegar
- 1 tsp Dijon mustard
- 1 tsp maple syrup
- Salt and pepper to taste

Instructions:

1. Preheat oven to 400°F. Wrap the beets in foil and roast for 45•60 minutes, until tender when pierced with a fork. Allow to cool, then peel and dice the beets.

2. In a large salad bowl, combine the arugula, diced beets, and chopped walnuts.

3. In a small bowl, whisk together the olive oil, balsamic vinegar, Dijon mustard, and maple syrup. Season with salt and pepper.

4. Drizzle the dressing over the salad and toss gently to coat.

5. Top the salad with the crumbled feta cheese, if using.

6. Serve immediately. Enjoy!

The key menopause•friendly ingredients in this recipe are:

- Arugula • a nutrient•dense leafy green that is high in calcium and folate
- Beets • a root vegetable rich in phytoestrogens and antioxidants
- Walnuts • a good source of omega•3 fatty acids, which can help reduce inflammation
- Maple syrup • a natural sweetener that is lower in glycemic index than refined sugar

This salad is a great source of fiber, vitamins, and minerals that can help support women during menopause. The combination of the peppery arugula, sweet beets, and crunchy walnuts makes for a delicious and nutritious meal.

103. Kale and Quinoa Salad

Ingredient:

- 1 cup uncooked quinoa, rinsed
- 2 cups vegetable broth or water
- 1 bunch kale, stems removed and leaves chopped
- 1 cup cherry tomatoes, halved
- 1 cucumber, diced
- 1/2 cup crumbled feta cheese (optional)
- 1/4 cup toasted sliced almonds
- 2 tbsp olive oil
- 2 tbsp lemon juice
- 1 tbsp Dijon mustard
- 1 tsp honey or maple syrup
- Salt and pepper to taste

Instructions:

1. In a medium saucepan, combine the quinoa and vegetable broth (or water). Bring to a boil, then reduce heat to low, cover and simmer for 15•20 minutes, until quinoa is cooked through. Fluff with a fork and set aside to cool.

2. In a large salad bowl, combine the chopped kale, cherry tomatoes, diced cucumber, crumbled feta (if using), and toasted almonds.

3. In a small bowl, whisk together the olive oil, lemon juice, Dijon mustard, and honey or maple syrup. Season with salt and pepper.

4. Add the cooked and cooled quinoa to the salad bowl. Drizzle the dressing over the salad and toss gently to coat.

5. Let the salad sit for 5•10 minutes to allow the kale to soften slightly. Serve chilled or at room temperature.

This kale and quinoa salad is packed with nutrients, protein, and fiber. The combination of the hearty kale, fluffy quinoa, fresh veggies, and tangy dressing makes for a delicious and satisfying meal. Enjoy!

104. Cucumber and Tomato Salad with Mint

Ingredient:

- 2 medium cucumbers, sliced
- 2 cups cherry or grape tomatoes, halved
- 1/2 red onion, thinly sliced
- 1/4 cup chopped fresh mint leaves
- 2 tbsp olive oil
- 2 tbsp red wine vinegar
- 1 tsp Dijon mustard
- 1 tsp honey (or maple syrup for vegan)
- 1/4 tsp salt
- 1/8 tsp black pepper

Instructions:

1. In a large bowl, combine the sliced cucumbers, halved tomatoes, and thinly sliced red onion.

2. In a small bowl, whisk together the olive oil, red wine vinegar, Dijon mustard, honey (or maple syrup), salt, and black pepper to make the dressing.

3. Pour the dressing over the cucumber and tomato mixture. Toss gently to coat.

4. Sprinkle the chopped fresh mint leaves over the salad and toss again lightly.

5. Cover and refrigerate the salad for at least 30 minutes to allow the flavors to meld.

6. Serve the chilled cucumber and tomato salad with mint.

Variations:
- Add crumbled feta or goat cheese for extra flavor.
- Swap the red onion for thinly sliced shallot.
- Use a combination of cherry tomatoes and diced beefsteak tomatoes.
- Stir in some diced avocado just before serving.
- Garnish with toasted pine nuts or sliced almonds.

This refreshing cucumber and tomato salad with fresh mint is the perfect light and healthy side dish. The tangy vinaigrette complements the crisp veggies beautifully. Enjoy it on its own or alongside grilled proteins, sandwiches, or Mediterranean•inspired meals.

105. Roasted Vegetable Salad with Tahini Dressing

Ingredient:

For the Roasted Vegetables:
- 1 medium sweet potato, peeled and cubed
- 1 red bell pepper, chopped
- 1 zucchini, chopped
- 1 red onion, sliced
- 2 tbsp olive oil
- Salt and pepper to taste

For the Salad:
- 5 oz mixed greens
- 1 cup cooked quinoa
- 1/4 cup toasted pumpkin seeds

For the Tahini Dressing:
- 1/4 cup tahini
- 2 tbsp lemon juice
- 1 tbsp maple syrup
- 1 garlic clove, minced
- 2•3 tbsp water, to thin
- Salt and pepper to taste

Instructions:

1. Preheat oven to 400°F. Toss the cubed sweet potato, bell pepper, zucchini, and onion with the olive oil on a large baking sheet. Season with salt and pepper.

2. Roast the vegetables for 20•25 minutes, stirring halfway, until tender and lightly browned.

3. In a large salad bowl, combine the mixed greens, cooked quinoa, and toasted pumpkin seeds.

4. In a small bowl, whisk together the tahini, lemon juice, maple syrup, and garlic. Add water 1 tbsp at a time to thin the dressing to your desired consistency. Season with salt and pepper.

5. Add the roasted vegetables to the salad bowl. Drizzle the tahini dressing over the top and toss gently to coat.

6. Serve the roasted vegetable salad immediately. Enjoy!

This salad is packed with nutrient•dense vegetables, protein•rich quinoa, and a creamy tahini dressing. The combination of flavors and textures makes for a delicious and satisfying meal.

106. Mixed Greens with Pomegranate Seeds

Ingredient:

- 5 oz mixed greens (such as spinach, arugula, kale)
- 1/2 cup pomegranate seeds
- 1/4 cup toasted sliced almonds
- 2 tbsp crumbled feta cheese (optional)
- 2 tbsp olive oil
- 1 tbsp balsamic vinegar
- 1 tsp Dijon mustard
- 1 tsp honey
- Salt and pepper to taste

Instructions:

1. In a large salad bowl, combine the mixed greens, pomegranate seeds, toasted almonds, and crumbled feta (if using).

2. In a small bowl, whisk together the olive oil, balsamic vinegar, Dijon mustard, and honey. Season with salt and pepper.

3. Drizzle the dressing over the salad and toss gently to coat.

4. Serve the mixed greens salad immediately.

This salad is a beautiful and nutritious combination of fresh greens, sweet pomegranate seeds, and crunchy almonds. The tangy balsamic•Dijon dressing complements the other flavors perfectly.

Some of the key benefits of this salad:

- Mixed greens are packed with vitamins, minerals, and antioxidants.
- Pomegranate seeds are a great source of fiber, vitamins, and antioxidants.
- Almonds provide healthy fats, protein, and fiber.
- Feta cheese (if using) adds a creamy, tangy element.

This salad makes for a light yet satisfying meal or side dish. The vibrant colors and flavors make it a great option for any occasion.

107. Thai Mango Salad

Ingredient:

- 2 ripe mangoes, peeled and sliced
- 2 cups shredded red cabbage
- 1 cup shredded carrots
- 1/2 cup chopped fresh cilantro
- 1/4 cup chopped roasted peanuts
- 2 tbsp lime juice
- 1 tbsp rice vinegar
- 1 tbsp sesame oil
- 1 tsp maple syrup
- 1 tsp grated ginger
- 1/4 tsp red pepper flakes (optional)
- Salt and pepper to taste

Instructions:

1. In a large salad bowl, combine the sliced mangoes, shredded red cabbage, shredded carrots, and chopped cilantro.

2. In a small bowl, whisk together the lime juice, rice vinegar, sesame oil, maple syrup, grated ginger, and red pepper flakes (if using). Season with salt and pepper.

3. Drizzle the dressing over the salad and toss gently to coat.

4. Sprinkle the chopped roasted peanuts over the top of the salad.

5. Serve immediately, or refrigerate for 30 minutes to allow the flavors to meld.

The key menopause•friendly ingredients in this recipe are:

- Mangoes • a tropical fruit rich in vitamins, minerals, and antioxidants
- Ginger • has anti•inflammatory properties that can help with menopause symptoms
- Maple syrup • a natural sweetener that is lower in glycemic index than refined sugar
- Peanuts • a good source of protein, fiber, and healthy fats

This refreshing and flavorful salad is a great way to incorporate more plant•based, nutrient•dense foods into your diet during menopause. The combination of sweet mango, crunchy vegetables, and a tangy•sweet dressing makes for a delicious and satisfying meal.

108. Watermelon and Feta Salad (with Tofu Feta)

Ingredient:

For the Tofu Feta:
- 1 block extra•firm tofu, pressed and cubed
- 2 tbsp lemon juice
- 1 tbsp apple cider vinegar
- 1 tsp dried oregano
- 1/2 tsp salt

For the Salad:
- 4 cups cubed watermelon
- 1 cup cherry tomatoes, halved
- 1/2 cup fresh basil leaves, chopped
- 2 tbsp olive oil
- 1 tbsp balsamic glaze
- Salt and pepper to taste

Instructions:

1. Make the tofu feta: In a small bowl, combine the cubed tofu, lemon juice, apple cider vinegar, oregano, and salt. Toss gently to coat. Cover and refrigerate for at least 30 minutes to allow the flavors to develop.

2. In a large salad bowl, combine the cubed watermelon, cherry tomatoes, and chopped basil.

3. Drizzle the olive oil and balsamic glaze over the salad and toss gently to coat.

4. Gently fold in the marinated tofu feta cubes.

5. Season the salad with salt and pepper to taste.

6. Serve immediately or refrigerate until ready to serve.

The key menopause•friendly ingredients in this recipe are:

- Watermelon • a hydrating fruit that is rich in vitamins, minerals, and antioxidants
- Tofu • a plant•based protein that can help with bone health during menopause
- Basil • an herb that contains compounds that may help alleviate hot flashes
- Balsamic glaze • a reduced balsamic vinegar that is lower in sugar than regular balsamic

This refreshing and flavorful salad is a great way to enjoy the sweetness of watermelon and the tanginess of the tofu feta. The combination of the juicy fruit, fresh herbs, and balsamic dressing makes for a delicious and nutritious menopause•friendly meal.

109. Chickpea and Avocado Salad

Ingredient:

- 1 (15 oz) can chickpeas, drained and rinsed
- 1 ripe avocado, diced
- 1/2 cup diced cucumber
- 1/4 cup diced red onion
- 2 tbsp chopped fresh cilantro
- 2 tbsp lime juice
- 1 tbsp olive oil
- 1 tsp Dijon mustard
- 1 tsp maple syrup
- Salt and pepper to taste

Instructions:

1. In a large bowl, gently toss together the chickpeas, diced avocado, cucumber, red onion, and chopped cilantro.

2. In a small bowl, whisk together the lime juice, olive oil, Dijon mustard, and maple syrup. Season with salt and pepper.

3. Drizzle the dressing over the chickpea and avocado salad and toss gently to coat.

4. Serve immediately or refrigerate for 30 minutes to allow the flavors to meld.

The key menopause•friendly ingredients in this recipe are:

- Chickpeas • a good source of plant•based protein, fiber, and complex carbohydrates
- Avocado • rich in healthy fats, vitamins, and minerals that can help with hormone balance
- Cilantro • an herb that may help alleviate hot flashes and other menopause symptoms
- Maple syrup • a natural sweetener that is lower in glycemic index than refined sugar

This salad is a nutritious and satisfying meal that can help support women during menopause. The combination of protein•rich chickpeas, creamy avocado, and fresh vegetables makes for a delicious and filling dish. Enjoy!

110. Mediterranean Farro Salad

Ingredient:

- 1 cup dry farro, cooked according to package instructions
- 1 cup diced cucumber
- 1 cup cherry tomatoes, halved
- 1/2 cup kalamata olives, pitted and halved
- 1/4 cup chopped fresh parsley
- 2 tbsp chopped fresh basil
- 2 tbsp olive oil
- 2 tbsp lemon juice
- 1 tbsp red wine vinegar
- 1 tsp Dijon mustard
- 1 tsp maple syrup
- 1 clove garlic, minced
- Salt and pepper to taste

Instructions:

1. Cook the farro according to package instructions. Drain and let cool.

2. In a large bowl, combine the cooked and cooled farro, diced cucumber, cherry tomatoes, kalamata olives, chopped parsley, and chopped basil.

3. In a small bowl, whisk together the olive oil, lemon juice, red wine vinegar, Dijon mustard, maple syrup, and minced garlic. Season with salt and pepper.

4. Drizzle the dressing over the farro salad and toss gently to coat.

5. Refrigerate for at least 30 minutes to allow the flavors to meld. Serve chilled or at room temperature.

The key menopause•friendly ingredients in this recipe are:

- Farro • a whole grain that is high in fiber, protein, and minerals
- Olives • a source of healthy fats and antioxidants
- Parsley • an herb that may help alleviate hot flashes
- Basil • an herb that contains compounds that may help with hormone balance
- Maple syrup • a natural sweetener that is lower in glycemic index than refined sugar

This Mediterranean•inspired farro salad is a delicious and nutritious option for women during menopause. The combination of whole grains, fresh vegetables, and a tangy dressing makes for a satisfying and flavorful meal.

111. Mediterranean Buddha Bowl

Ingredient:

- 1 cup cooked quinoa
- 1 cup roasted chickpeas
- 1 cup chopped cucumber
- 1 cup cherry tomatoes, halved
- 1/2 cup kalamata olives, pitted and halved
- 1/4 cup crumbled feta cheese (optional)
- 2 tbsp chopped fresh parsley
- 2 tbsp olive oil
- 1 tbsp red wine vinegar
- 1 tsp Dijon mustard
- 1 tsp maple syrup
- 1 clove garlic, minced
- Salt and pepper to taste

Instructions:

1. Prepare the quinoa according to package instructions. Set aside to cool.

2. Preheat oven to 400°F. Toss the chickpeas with 1 tbsp of olive oil and season with salt and pepper. Roast for 15•20 minutes, until crispy.

3. In a large bowl, combine the cooked quinoa, roasted chickpeas, chopped cucumber, cherry tomatoes, kalamata olives, and crumbled feta (if using).

4. In a small bowl, whisk together the remaining 1 tbsp olive oil, red wine vinegar, Dijon mustard, maple syrup, and minced garlic. Season with salt and pepper. Drizzle the dressing over the buddha bowl and toss gently to coat.

6. Sprinkle the chopped parsley over the top. Serve immediately or refrigerate until ready to enjoy.

The key menopause•friendly ingredients in this recipe are:

- Quinoa • a high•protein, high•fiber grain that can help with weight management
- Chickpeas • a good source of plant•based protein and fiber
- Olives • a source of healthy fats and antioxidants
- Parsley • an herb that may help alleviate hot flashes
- Maple syrup • a natural sweetener lower in glycemic index than refined sugar

112. Mexican Rice Bowl with Black Beans

Ingredient:

- 1 cup cooked brown rice
- 1 (15 oz) can black beans, drained and rinsed
- 1 cup diced tomatoes
- 1/2 cup diced red onion
- 1/2 cup diced bell pepper
- 2 tbsp chopped fresh cilantro
- 1 tbsp lime juice
- 1 tsp ground cumin
- 1 tsp chili powder
- 1 tsp maple syrup
- Salt and pepper to taste
- Sliced avocado, for serving

Instructions:

1. In a large bowl, combine the cooked brown rice, black beans, diced tomatoes, red onion, bell pepper, and chopped cilantro.

2. In a small bowl, whisk together the lime juice, cumin, chili powder, and maple syrup. Season with salt and pepper.

3. Drizzle the dressing over the rice and bean mixture and toss gently to coat.

4. Serve the Mexican rice bowl topped with sliced avocado.

The key menopause•friendly ingredients in this recipe are:

- Brown rice • a whole grain that is high in fiber and B vitamins
- Black beans • a good source of plant•based protein and fiber
- Avocado • a healthy fat that can help with hormone balance
- Cilantro • an herb that may help alleviate hot flashes and other menopause symptoms
- Maple syrup • a natural sweetener that is lower in glycemic index than refined sugar

This Mexican•inspired rice bowl is a nutritious and satisfying meal that can help support women during menopause. The combination of whole grains, legumes, vegetables, and healthy fats makes it a well•balanced and nourishing dish.

113. Sushi Bowl with Seaweed and Avocado

Ingredient:

- 1 cup cooked brown rice
- 1 cup shredded carrots
- 1 cup shredded cucumber
- 1 ripe avocado, sliced
- 1/2 cup shredded nori sheets (seaweed)
- 2 tbsp toasted sesame seeds
- 2 tbsp rice vinegar
- 1 tbsp soy sauce or tamari
- 1 tsp sesame oil
- 1 tsp maple syrup
- 1 tsp grated ginger
- Salt and pepper to taste

Instructions:

1. In a large bowl, combine the cooked brown rice, shredded carrots, shredded cucumber, sliced avocado, and shredded nori sheets.

2. In a small bowl, whisk together the rice vinegar, soy sauce, sesame oil, maple syrup, and grated ginger. Season with salt and pepper.

3. Drizzle the dressing over the sushi bowl and toss gently to coat.

4. Sprinkle the toasted sesame seeds over the top.

5. Serve immediately or refrigerate until ready to enjoy.

The key menopause•friendly ingredients in this recipe are:

- Brown rice • a whole grain that is high in fiber and B vitamins
- Nori sheets • a type of seaweed that is a good source of iodine and other minerals
- Avocado • a healthy fat that can help with hormone balance
- Ginger • has anti•inflammatory properties that can help with menopause symptoms
- Maple syrup • a natural sweetener that is lower in glycemic index than refined sugar

This sushi•inspired bowl is a delicious and nutritious meal that can help support women during menopause. The combination of whole grains, fresh vegetables, healthy fats, and nutrient•dense seaweed makes it a well•balanced and satisfying dish.

114. Thai Curry Bowl with Tofu

Ingredient:

- 1 block extra•firm tofu, cubed
- 1 tbsp coconut oil
- 1 cup cooked brown rice
- 1 cup chopped broccoli florets
- 1 cup sliced mushrooms
- 1/2 cup diced red bell pepper
- 1/4 cup chopped green onions
- 2 tbsp chopped fresh cilantro
- 2 tbsp Thai red curry paste
- 1 cup coconut milk
- 1 tsp grated ginger
- 1 tsp maple syrup
- Salt and pepper to taste

Instructions:

1. In a large skillet, heat the coconut oil over medium heat. Add the cubed tofu and sauté for 5•7 minutes, until lightly browned on all sides. Remove tofu from the pan and set aside.

2. In the same skillet, add the chopped broccoli, sliced mushrooms, and diced bell pepper. Sauté for 3•4 minutes, until vegetables are tender.

3. Stir in the Thai red curry paste and coconut milk. Bring the mixture to a simmer and cook for 2•3 minutes, until slightly thickened.

4. Add the sautéed tofu, chopped green onions, and grated ginger to the skillet. Simmer for an additional 2•3 minutes.

5. Remove from heat and stir in the maple syrup. Season with salt and pepper to taste.

6. To serve, divide the cooked brown rice into bowls and top with the Thai curry vegetable and tofu mixture. Garnish with chopped fresh cilantro.

This flavorful Thai curry bowl is a delicious and nutritious meal that can help support women during menopause. The combination of protein•rich tofu, fiber•rich vegetables, and aromatic spices makes for a satisfying and nourishing dish.

115. BBQ Tempeh Bowl with Coleslaw

Ingredient:

For the BBQ Tempeh:
- 8 oz tempeh, cut into cubes
- 1/2 cup BBQ sauce (look for one low in sugar)
- 1 tbsp olive oil

For the Coleslaw:
- 2 cups shredded green cabbage
- 1 cup shredded red cabbage
- 1 carrot, grated
- 2 tbsp apple cider vinegar
- 1 tbsp olive oil
- 1 tsp Dijon mustard
- 1 tsp maple syrup
- Salt and pepper to taste

For the Bowl:
- 1 cup cooked quinoa
- 1 avocado, sliced
- 2 tbsp toasted pumpkin seeds

Instructions:

1. Preheat oven to 400°F. Toss the tempeh cubes with the BBQ sauce and olive oil. Spread on a baking sheet and roast for 20•25 minutes, flipping halfway, until heated through and slightly crispy.

2. In a large bowl, combine the shredded green and red cabbage, grated carrot, apple cider vinegar, olive oil, Dijon mustard, and maple syrup. Season with salt and pepper. Toss to coat.

3. To assemble the bowls, start with a base of cooked quinoa. Top with the roasted BBQ tempeh, coleslaw, sliced avocado, and toasted pumpkin seeds.

This BBQ tempeh bowl with coleslaw is a nutritious and satisfying meal that can help support women during menopause. The combination of plant•based protein, fiber•rich vegetables, and healthy fats makes it a well•balanced and nourishing dish.

116. Mediterranean Couscous Bowl

Ingredient:

- 1 cup dry couscous, cooked according to package instructions
- 1 cup diced cucumber
- 1 cup cherry tomatoes, halved
- 1/2 cup kalamata olives, pitted and halved
- 1/4 cup crumbled feta cheese (optional)
- 2 tbsp chopped fresh parsley
- 2 tbsp chopped fresh basil
- 2 tbsp olive oil
- 2 tbsp lemon juice
- 1 tbsp red wine vinegar
- 1 tsp Dijon mustard
- 1 tsp maple syrup
- 1 clove garlic, minced
- Salt and pepper to taste

Instructions:

1. Cook the couscous according to package instructions. Fluff with a fork and let cool.

2. In a large bowl, combine the cooked couscous, diced cucumber, cherry tomatoes, kalamata olives, crumbled feta (if using), chopped parsley, and chopped basil.

3. In a small bowl, whisk together the olive oil, lemon juice, red wine vinegar, Dijon mustard, maple syrup, and minced garlic. Season with salt and pepper.

4. Drizzle the dressing over the couscous salad and toss gently to coat.

5. Refrigerate for at least 30 minutes to allow the flavors to meld.

6. Serve chilled or at room temperature.

This Mediterranean•inspired couscous bowl is a delicious and nutritious option for women during menopause. The combination of whole grains, fresh vegetables, and a tangy dressing makes for a satisfying and flavorful meal.

117. Protein·Packed Lentil Bowl

Ingredient:

- 1 cup cooked brown lentils
- 1 cup cooked quinoa
- 1 cup roasted sweet potato cubes
- 1 cup sautéed spinach
- 1/2 cup diced avocado
- 2 tbsp toasted pumpkin seeds
- 2 tbsp tahini
- 1 tbsp lemon juice
- 1 tsp maple syrup
- 1 clove garlic, minced
- Salt and pepper to taste

Instructions:

1. In a large bowl, combine the cooked brown lentils, cooked quinoa, roasted sweet potato cubes, and sautéed spinach.

2. In a small bowl, whisk together the tahini, lemon juice, maple syrup, and minced garlic. Season with salt and pepper.

3. Drizzle the tahini dressing over the lentil and quinoa bowl and toss gently to coat.

4. Top the bowl with the diced avocado and toasted pumpkin seeds. Serve immediately, or refrigerate until ready to enjoy.

The key menopause·friendly ingredients in this recipe are:

- Lentils · a high·protein, high·fiber legume that can help with weight management
- Quinoa · a complete protein that is also high in fiber and minerals
- Sweet potato · a nutrient·dense root vegetable that is rich in beta·carotene
- Spinach · a leafy green that is high in calcium and folate
- Avocado · a healthy fat that can help with hormone balance
- Pumpkin seeds · a good source of zinc, which is important for menopausal women
- Tahini · a sesame seed paste that is rich in calcium

This protein·packed lentil bowl is a nutritious and satisfying meal that can help support women during menopause. The combination of plant·based proteins, complex carbohydrates, healthy fats, and nutrient·dense vegetables makes it a well·balanced and nourishing dish.

Congratulations on completing ***"115+ Vegan Recipes for Menopause Health and Happiness"!*** By exploring these recipes and incorporating plant-based nutrition into your lifestyle, you have taken a significant step toward enhancing your health and well-being during menopause.

Reflecting on the Journey

This journey has been about more than just food. It's been about embracing a new phase of life with positivity and proactive health choices. Menopause can bring challenges, but it also offers an opportunity to reassess and redefine your health priorities. Through these 115+ recipes, you've discovered the power of plant-based nutrition to support hormone balance, boost energy levels, and promote overall vitality.

Celebrating Plant-Based Nutrition

The benefits of a vegan diet during menopause are profound. From reducing the risk of chronic diseases to improving mood and supporting bone health, plant-based foods provide the essential nutrients your body needs. By choosing a variety of colorful fruits, vegetables, grains, legumes, nuts, and seeds, you're nourishing your body with nature's best offerings.

Looking Forward

As you move forward, continue to experiment with new recipes and ingredients. Let this cookbook be a foundation for your culinary adventures, but don't be afraid to innovate and create your own plant-based masterpieces. Share these meals with family and friends, spreading the joy and benefits of vegan living.

Maintaining Balance

Remember, wellness is about balance. Alongside a nutritious diet, prioritize regular physical activity, adequate rest, and mindfulness practices. Listen to your body's needs and honor them with self-care and compassion.

Thank You

Thank you for embarking on this culinary journey with us. We hope these recipes have brought joy to your kitchen and nourishment to your body. May you continue to thrive, finding health and happiness in every meal and moment.

Here's to a vibrant and fulfilling menopause journey!

With heartfelt gratitude,